Lung Cancer Chronicles

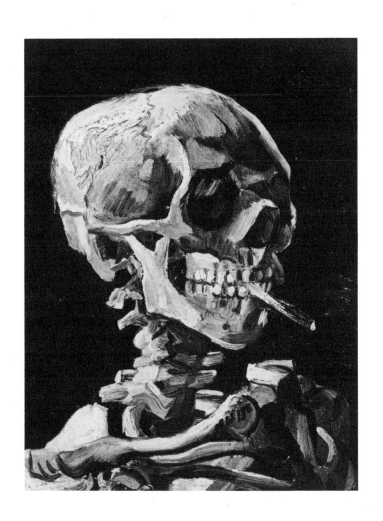

LUNG CANCER CHRONICLES

John A. Meyer, M.D.

RUTGERS UNIVERSITY PRESS

New Brunswick and London

Frontispiece. Vincent van Gogh, Skull with Cigarette (1886). Oil on canvas. Collection Vincent van Gogh Foundation/National Museum Vincent van Gogh, Amsterdam.

Epigraph to chapter 16 copyright 1986 by Time Inc. All rights reserved. Reprinted by permission from TIME.

Library of Congress Cataloging-in-Publication Data
Meyer, John A., 1927–
Lung cancer chronicles / John A. Meyer.
p.   cm.
Includes bibliographical references.
ISBN 0-8135-1492-4 (cloth)   ISBN 0-8135-1493-2 (pbk.)
1. Lungs—Cancer—Popular works.   2. Tobacco habit—Health
aspects.   I. Title.
[DNLM: 1. Lung Neoplasms.   2. Patient Education.   3. Smoking—
adverse effects.   WF 658 M612L]
RC280.L8M49   1990
616.99'424—dc20
DNLM   /DLC
for Library of Congress   89-11000
CIP

British Cataloging-in-Publication
information available

FOR M.A., BILL, JOHN, AND NINA

I lived through the whole war, being of an age to
comprehend events, and giving my attention to them
in order to know the exact truth about them.

—Thucydides (c. 462–c. 404 B.C.), *History of
the Peloponnesian War* 5.26

Contents

Preface

Announcer: Ladies and gentlemen, the late Mr. Yul Brynner.

Mr. Brynner: I really wanted to make a commercial when I discovered that I was that sick, and my time was so limited. To make a commercial that says, simply, "Now that I'm gone, I tell you, *Don't smoke.* Whatever you do, *just don't smoke.*" If I could take back that smoking, I wouldn't be talking about any cancer. I'm convinced of that.

—Yul Brynner (1920–1985), in a tape made for release after his death. Courtesy of the American Cancer Society, Inc.

The topic of lung cancer is not cheerful or optimistic. Does the public need or even wish to know more about it? After all, we all hope it will never concern us. If all of us knew more about it, would not the disease be less able to afflict us? Medical textbooks are dry, ponderous, incomprehensible, and of forbidding length because they need to include everything, like encyclopedias. They are also largely inaccessible except to physicians. This chronicle was undertaken in the hope that the problem of lung cancer could be clarified for the sake of interest as well as understanding, and in language that we all understand. Three short appendices at the end discuss some technical aspects in more detail, for those readers who might be especially interested. The appendices could equally well be skipped over. A glossary has sought to define any terms with which the nonmedical reader may not be familiar.

Human behavior in accordance with intelligent self-interest, unfortunately, remains difficult for us all. Death from lung cancer is the needless calamity; in 85 to 90 percent of cases, it would never have occurred if the person had not smoked. Yet lung cancer is by far the leading cause of cancer deaths in our society. Hardly any of us are able to believe that the ultimate disaster can ever strike ourselves.

Lung cancer would not be such a disaster if the medical profession were able to treat it with fairly routine hope of cure; unfortunately, such is not the case, and we must examine the issue in detail. Segments of the public dislike the medical profession for a variety of reasons, some perhaps deserved, others possibly not. But the profession no longer says, "Do as I say, not as I do." Hardly any physicians smoke today, and practically all urge abstinence from smoking on their patients as strongly as possible. Could it be that the medical profession understands that a dramatic and reliable "cure" is unlikely during any of our lifetimes? We must plan to do without the long shot, the hundred-million-dollar lottery ticket. For this disease, we should need no more breakthroughs or Nobel Prizes, because we know already how the death rate from it could be cut by 85 percent. The public knows, too, because the profession has done its best to spread the word. But lung cancer will be with us for many years more.

Lung cancer patients named in this chronicle, and their physicians, all are fictitious except for public figures such as Yul Brynner and John Wayne. Any real or fancied resemblance of the hypothetical patients to persons living or dead can only be coincidental. The John C. Warren Memorial Hospital does not exist, for all that its real-life namesake (1778–1856) was Boston's foremost surgeon. Since this chronicle speaks to a collective audience, and not to an individual person, its words should not ever be relied upon above or in place of the advice of a personal physician.

J. M.
Syracuse, New York
April 1989

Lung Cancer Chronicles

One

IMPRINTING

Man is the only animal that laughs and weeps; for he
is the only animal that is struck by the difference
between what things are and what they ought to be.

—William Hazlitt (1778–1830)

AUGUST 1982

Terry alighted from the Green Line train at Museum station, crossed the
westbound lane of Huntington, and walked over to the museum's west
entrance. On this warm Saturday afternoon, she wore faded jeans, a
T-shirt, and sandals; she had slept late this morning and chose to spend
the afternoon enjoying her leisure. It would not last much longer; her
sophomore year at Aquinas High School was to begin in only a couple of
weeks. Outside the entrance to the new west wing Terry sat down on a
bench, relaxed, and pulled from her pocket the pack of Virginia Slims
with a book of matches. A photographer from the *Globe,* looking around
the park that afternoon for summer mood pictures, saw her sitting deep
in thought and recorded the moment visually. The picture appeared
Monday in the Metro section with the caption, "EASY DAY. Terry Barton, 15, enjoying the weekend sunshine on Saturday outside the Museum
of Fine Arts."

Neither the photographer, the caption writer, nor the city editor were
inclined to comment that the fifteen-year-old girl was smoking like a
veteran. Hardly any readers seeing the picture gave it a second thought;
you saw the same thing every day, whichever way you looked, and
anyway was it not a matter of her own free choice? Lots of teenaged boys
were smoking too.

JULY 1948

Reveille sounded at 6:00 A.M. over a single loudspeaker at the U.S. Forest Service work camp in the mountains of northern Idaho. Bill Hunter awoke with a start, cringing as usual at the shock of exposure to a damp, cold morning. The climate here deep in the forest didn't match one bit with his ideas of summer. Thirty-one other young men were struggling out of sleeping bags at the same time, jumping into clothes and jackets with their teeth chattering, some with uncontrollable shivers. Most were college students on summer employment, with a mix of migrant workers and transients, plus the ranger and his assistant who supervised the camp. All were here because of the Forest Service's effort to control the spreading blight of the white pine blister-rust disease.

Bill looked outside the tent flap after struggling into his clothes. The day was raw, wet, and cloudy with a steady drizzle from the skies. Nothing whatever warned him that this day would affect the rest of his life. He splashed water over his face from the wash trough in the lavatory tent; shaving was too much trouble here and he was letting his beard grow, for the first time in his life. But in the mess tent there were piles of flapjacks with butter and syrup, bacon, and mugs of steaming coffee. Breakfast began to bring him to life, and soon he believed that he might survive.

Out in the forest, lengths of white cloth tape had been stretched between trees as base line markers. The squads of men formed up in line at the point where work had ended the day before. Maintaining a distance of two yards from each man to the next, they moved slowly through the forest examining every foot of ground for wild gooseberry bushes, up-rooting every bush or sprout that could be found. The forest here was made up largely of majestic white pines, and the trees were being threatened with destruction by the fungus disease called blister rust. Control of the pest would never be possible if the fungus spread directly from tree to tree. But fungi have strange life histories; some live their existence in one form, then beget offspring of a completely different form which must infect an alternate host in order to survive. Wild gooseberry bushes had been found to be the alternate hosts; it was argued that if they could be eradicated from the pine forests, the blister-rust disease could no longer spread to healthy pine trees. No one knew, yet, whether such control actually would be possible, but the Forest Service had selected areas in several national forests for a test which would run for several years.

On this raw, drizzly day, the forest undergrowth was soaking wet.

Simply pushing through it in the required direction brought repeated cold soakings, while uprooting any gooseberry plants added to the discomfort. Lunch break came at last, and the crew ate their soggy sandwiches under the best available sheltering trees. Bill Hunter was nonplused when one of his friends pulled out a pack of "tailor-made" cigarettes, offered him one, and lit it for him. Somehow, the cold and the wet made it natural to accept—a thing he never had done before. In fact, the cigarette was a distinct comfort on such a day, not at all a choking poison as he had often imagined. At the brief mid-afternoon rest break he accepted another, and without having realized anything, he already was securely hooked.

Bill was twenty-one that summer, having taken the job because of a need to work outdoors after the confinement of his first year in medical school. He and a buddy had hitch-hiked West after school had ended, and here they were. Bill's time in college had been irregular and spotty, overshadowed by the draft in the closing year of the war as he had approached age eighteen, and interrupted by his induction in June 1945. The Japanese surrender had come while he was still in basic training. Eventually he found himself being shipped to Germany with many other young draftees to maintain the Occupation. Bill had always despised the smell of cigarette smoke; he hadn't been able to stand it either in college or in the army, where cigarettes were inescapable and all the more offensive for being dirt cheap, only a nickel a pack in the post exchanges. The Occupation soldiers got a weekly ration of one carton apiece—ten packs of cigarettes which cost only fifty cents in all. He had been astounded to see the value that the poor threadbare German civilians placed on them; any menial task was gladly and quickly done for only a couple of cigarettes, while a pack was a gift almost beyond price. Smoking still had not tempted him, until the chance occurrence on that unusual day in Idaho. Around the camp, most of the work crew smoked "roll-your-owns" from pocket sacks of Bull Durham tobacco. Bull Durham was part of the mystique of the West in the days before Marlboro Country had been dreamed up. A regular cigarette, "tailor-made," was a distinct luxury and almost an item of conspicuous consumption.

SEPTEMBER 1980

Dr. Bill Hunter, well into middle age, still was addicted to cigarettes as a result of that fateful day in 1948. Back in 1948, no studies had warned of the cumulative lethal hazards of smoking; in fact, during the late forties one cigarette company claimed preference for its product by the medical profession. "More Doctors Smoke Camels Than Any Other Cigarette!" shouted the ads and the billboards, showing an obviously eminent and successful physician lighting up or inhaling deeply. At about the end of Bill's third year in medical school, in 1950, a warning of real danger appeared in a paper in the *Journal of the American Medical Association*. The authors, a world-renowned professor of surgery and one of his medical students, found that almost all patients with lung cancer had been long-time heavy cigarette smokers; lung cancer rarely occurred in nonsmokers.[1] Their report strikes the reader today as oddly tentative, and unfortunately its shocking message went unheeded by too many smokers including many of those physicians who smoked. To be fair, the report of Wynder and Graham stood alone when first published, unsupported by the many statistical reviews which have appeared since then.

For eight years after his graduation from medical school, Bill had been immersed in residency training. There had been five years in general surgery, then a year on a research fellowship, then two additional years in thoracic surgery, surgery of the chest. The long hours, confinement, and fatigue of residency were a continual stress; and he never could break the smoking habit in spite of his increasing awareness of its dangers. Thoracic surgery, then as now, concerned itself with the first-line treatment of lung cancer; in the years since then, open heart surgery and eventually coronary artery bypass have taken up a very large part of the specialty. The epidemic of lung cancer in men was in its period of explosive growth, which now shows signs of leveling off. The newer epidemic among women had not yet made its appearance. Soon after the end of his training, Bill managed to quit smoking and abstained for a year. The craving for cigarettes never really disappeared. He fell easily into the trap that has snared so many smokers, the belief that after a year's abstinence he could take them or leave them alone. Unfortunately it simply was not possible to "leave them alone" while permitting himself to "take" them; and shortly he was more securely hooked than ever.

Bill was ready for a change of scene. A couple of years after completion of his residency training, he accepted the offer of a full-time faculty position as assistant professor of surgery at another medical school, this one located in Boston. He was destined to spend the rest of his professional life there. With obligations of teaching, and the need to pursue research studies as part of an academic career, his practice of thoracic surgery developed only slowly. Treatment of lung cancer remained the greatest challenge; surgery as a sole treatment was approaching the limits of its usefulness except for gradual refinements in anesthesia, postoperative care, and diagnostic methods.

In 1962 Dr. Luther Terry, surgeon general of the U.S. Public Health Service, appointed an advisory panel of physicians who in 1964 submitted the famous report *Smoking and Health*.[2] The report indicted cigarette smoking as the principal cause of the lung cancer epidemic in men (the epidemic had not really begun among women at the time, making its appearance about 1965), and a contributing cause of much chronic lung disease. Known ever since as "The Surgeon General's Report," the document was impressive for its reasoned analysis and the authority of its statements. Many subsequent reports have appeared from the surgeon general's office,[3] but the original has remained a landmark, more recently an obstacle to litigation against the tobacco companies by present-day smokers, since it was issued a quarter of a century ago.

Bitterly aware of the dangers of smoking, Bill tried several more times to quit but was unable to overcome the craving. Worst of all was the sense of intellectual dishonesty, of the need to tell patients to quit smoking when he was unable to do it himself. He could not abide the knowledge that some of his patients, lay people, had kicked the habit successfully while he, a physician and, worse, a thoracic surgeon, had been unable to do it. Disgust with himself finally built up to the point at which he came home from the hospital one Saturday afternoon in September, crushed up his two remaining packs of cigarettes, and threw them into the garbage can. This time, bitter and disgusted, he would not allow the craving to begin; he sustained his resolve with the angry question "Who needs it?"

In the following months he began to feel more alive again. The smoker's cough diminished, his breathing improved, and in a surprisingly short time he felt no craving at all for the habit. Food never had tasted so good as it did now; and like others who have quit, he had the difficult problem of weight control. The smell of cigarette smoke became distinctly offensive once more; every day it was easier to maintain his resolve. Oddly, though he no longer felt any craving, and in fact never touched a cigarette again, for years after quitting he continued to dream that he had been smoking. In the dream, his painfully built-up habit of abstinence had been washed away.

There remained the difficult and unanswered question: Had it been any better to quit late than not to have quit at all? Bill knew that to some degree at least, the cumulative lethal risk of smoking would continue to hang over him for the rest of his life. A number of careful statistical reviews had found a rapid decline in the risk of heart disease after quitting, heart disease being the greatest single threat of smoking-related premature death. There is, however, only a very gradual decline in the risk of lung cancer which never fully returns to the risk level of a lifelong nonsmoker. Better or not, he felt that it was the only thing he could have done, in order to regain at least a part of his personal integrity.

SEPTEMBER 1987

Terry Barton walked back to her room after the last afternoon class. She was a junior at the state university and literally moving up in the world; this year her room was on the twelfth floor of one of the new high-rise dormitories. There were some problems to go along with the view. In the two weeks since classes had started, the dormitory had been evacuated four times because of fire alarms, and she had had to run all the way down the crowded stair wells with everyone else. The prank alarms, if such they had been, were beginning to interfere with sleep as well as with studying.

She had been glad to come back this fall and immerse herself in her studies, because the summer had been a terrible and distressing one. From the start of college, Terry had planned her future as a high school art teacher, and this past spring she had declared her major accordingly. Already she was looking forward to a field trip in October to see the thirty-odd Renoirs, plus the Monets and Cézannes, at the spectacular little museum in Williamstown.

In May, Terry's mother had called from Florida to say that her dad would be entering the hospital in a few days for surgery; could she come right down? Dad's appearance had shocked her when she arrived. She had not understood that he had become seriously, even desperately, ill; he was only fifty-eight.

Kenneth Barton had retired as a chief petty officer after thirty years in the navy and returned home with his family to the Boston area. For five years he had worked in the Engineering and Maintenance department at the West Roxbury V. A. Hospital. He was having increasing trouble with shortness of breath; every winter there were several absentee periods when a cold or other respiratory infection would lay him low. He couldn't do without a couple of packs of cigarettes a day. Finally he gave up the job and moved to Sarasota with his wife. Terry was starting college, and her older brother was working in Waltham, so both stayed behind.

Since January of 1987 Ken had been losing weight—a total of almost forty pounds—and his cough had gradually grown worse. He was troubled by increasing weakness and easy fatigue. Ken had always stayed away from doctors, but this time his wife insisted that he see one. A chest x-ray showed an abnormal shadow in his right lung. Other tests followed: a test of his breathing capacity; scans of his chest and abdomen, brain, and bones; and a bronchoscopy or inspection of the interior of the bronchial passages through a slim, flexible fiberoptic scope. A tiny biopsy taken at this time had proved the diagnosis of lung cancer. The physician had a blunt and plain talk with him, saying in effect that the situation did not look good but that so far, no absolute indication of inoperability had been found. He wanted to arrange a consultation with a thoracic surgeon. The surgeon agreed, advising Ken that one all-out try for surgical removal seemed necessary. A date was set for hospital admission, with the surgery to be done the next day. Terry flew down on the day of his admission to the university hospital in Tampa.

On the day of the operation, Terry waited with her mother after Ken had been taken away, neither of them saying much. Eventually the surgeon returned, wearing a long white coat over his scrub suit; he was saying some things about the tumor being fixed, impossible to remove, something about radiation therapy. She hardly heard him but had the distinct impression that the message was bad.

Ken recovered slowly and was released from the hospital ten days after the operation. Before discharge, he was taken in a wheel chair for the first consultation with the radiotherapist, a soft-spoken Chinese physician with never-failing politeness and regard for Ken's feelings. He explained the plan of treatment: a short session in front of the cobalt unit every weekday; weekends off; treatments to continue for three weeks or possibly four, depending upon how Ken was tolerating them. A date was set for the first session, about two weeks after his discharge.

At home, it was difficult to get around much, or to increase his activity. Ken continued to lose weight, and the radiation treatments spoiled his appetite even more. The doctor had said this effect would pass off after treatment was finished. Having had no pain so far except for that caused by the operation, he noticed little change or improvement after the treatments. His cough persisted but could be controlled by the prescription medicine he had been given. On some days he was feverish and sweated a lot.

By August his condition was deteriorating again. In another frank discussion, his physician intimated that there might not be much time left. Chemotherapy was mentioned, but the doctor said plainly that it could offer little or no chance of benefit in this situation; he would not advise it. One evening when Terry's mother was out of the house, Ken confided some of his anguished fears to Terry, "I'm getting so weak that I'm afraid to go to sleep at night any more. Any one of these mornings I may not wake up again." In fact, it was only ten days later that he sank into a coma and expired within a few hours. For his family, the small funeral was a sad and lonely remembrance; afterward Terry could recall little of the Mass except the words about ashes to ashes and dust to dust.

Back at school now, Terry smoked as she always had. It was the thing young women did; it was inseparable from self-image; after all they had come a long way, as the advertisements said. More to the point, she could not get through a few hours, let alone a day or more, without having cigarettes within easy reach. The danger of premature death from lung cancer seemed impossibly remote at age twenty, and anyway, there always was subconscious reassurance that such a thing could not happen to her.

Dr. Bill Hunter never saw or met Terry Barton. The actuarial tables clearly ordained that he would be in retirement, or more probably dead, before there could be any chance that the unthinkable catastrophe might befall Terry as it had her father. But several years before, Bill had chanced to see the "Easy Day" picture in the *Globe* and he could not forget it; in fact, he had cut out the picture and saved it in his files. Just at that time, he had been approaching his anniversary of two years' abstinence and no longer had any trouble maintaining his resolve, but the picture of the pretty young girl with her cigarettes had been painful and distressing. In one second, it had brought back the time of his addiction and all of his problems in coping with it.

Two

EPIDEMIC

It addes to the affliction, that relapses are (and for the most part justly) imputed to our selves, as occasioned by some disorder in us; and so we are not onely passive, but active, in our own ruine; wee doe not onely stand under a falling house, but pull it downe upon us; and wee are not onely executed (that implies guiltinesse) but wee are executioners of our selves.

—John Donne, *Meditation XXIII* (1624)

The late Dr. Alton Ochsner of New Orleans (1896–1981), widely loved and honored as a surgeon, teacher, and pioneer, possessed insight and vision beyond that of most of his contemporaries. Long before the medical community had blamed lung cancer on smoking, and though hardly anyone was listening, he carried on a personal vendetta against the dangers of this newly popular habit. In his own words,

As a junior student in 1919 at Washington University, I recall vividly seeing a patient with cancer of the lung who was admitted to the Barnes Hospital. As is usual, the patient died. Dr. George Dock, our eminent professor of medicine, who was also a great pathologist, insisted upon having the junior and senior classes witness the autopsy because he said the condition was so rare that he thought we might never see another case. . . . I did not see another case until 1936, seventeen years later, when in a period of six months, I saw nine cases of cancer of the lung. Having been impressed with the extreme rarity of this condition seventeen years previously, this represented an epidemic for which there had to be a cause. All the afflicted patients were men who smoked heavily and had smoked since World War I. I then ascertained that cigarettes were consumed relatively infrequently until World War I but that during and following the war their use had greatly increased. Because of the parallelism between cigarette consumption and the increased incidence of lung cancer (with approximately a twenty-year lag), I had the temerity, at that time, to postulate that the probable cause of this new epidemic was cigarette use.[1]

In a posthumous tribute to Dr. Ochsner, his close friend and former associate Dr. Michael E. DeBakey also spoke of this insight: "He first speculated in 1936 that there was a causal relationship between smoking and carcinoma of the lung. It was then that he began a one-man crusade against cigarette smoking. The scientific proof, many years later, of that causal relationship gave witness to his vision."[2] Dr. Ochsner himself never conducted any statistical studies, being a surgeon and a man of action, but spoke with convictions derived from his own experience; for this reason such later careful analyses as the "Surgeon General's Report" are remembered as the landmarks that linked smoking to lung cancer. Dr. Ochsner preached his message with humor as well as conviction. Dr. Bill Hunter recalled the day, years before, that Dr. Ochsner had been invited as guest speaker at the Department of Surgery weekly conference while he (Bill) had been an assistant resident in surgery. Such a visiting speaker appeared a remote and Olympian figure to the young residents. Dr. Ochsner had made his closely reasoned presentation and spent fifteen minutes more answering questions from the audience. "Yes, but there is also another thing"; he added finally, "in babies born to mothers who have smoked heavily, if you look carefully down at the end of the spine, you will find a small butt!"

We are living in the midst of a lethal epidemic, needless and tragic, and for the most part preventable. Lung cancer has been the leading cause of cancer death among women in the United States since 1986, when it surpassed breast cancer; while among men in the United States, there is no other cancer that even approaches it as a killer. (In this discussion, we cannot deal with the other health hazards of smoking, among which are increased risk of heart attack, stroke, emphysema, and several other cancers. Lung cancer by itself is topic enough.) In vital statistics, "death rate" from a given cause is defined as the number of deaths from that cause, per 100,000 of population, per year, the population having been adjusted to the age distribution at the previous U.S. census for uniformity in comparison. Not only do the total number of deaths from lung cancer continue to increase from year to year (after all, the population continues

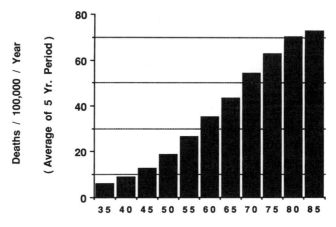

Figure 2.1. Chart of the lung cancer death rates among U. S. men, by five-year periods, 1930–1985. Source: *U. S. National Center for Health Statistics; Ref. 3–19).*

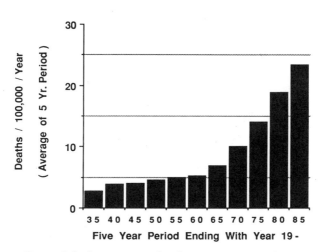

Figure 2.2. Chart of the lung cancer death rates among U. S. women, by five-year periods, 1930–1985. Source: *U. S. National Center for Health Statistics; Ref. 3–19).*

to increase), but the death rate per 100,000 continues to go up. The epidemic first made its appearance in men (fig. 2.1), since they were first to become addicted to the smoking habit. Many people, men in particular, have given up the habit in recent years; a partial break, or slowing, in the yearly increase of death rates among men is just becoming visible on the graphs.

For women, smoking still was widely regarded as socially unacceptable, at least until about the time of World War II; and lung cancer in women remained a rarity until the approximately twenty-year lag period after the war had begun to expire (fig. 2.2). Could it be that in this instance, women actually were benefited by "social injustice" and "repressive mores"? Now the epidemic among women is gaining rapidly. Women are by no means immune, and many studies suggest that they are less able to give up the habit, once acquired, than are men. No prospect can be seen of any slowing of the epidemic in women. The lung cancer death rate among women in the United States in 1985, the last year for which full statistics are available, was 26.6 per 100,000 per year compared to the five-year average of 23.3 (fig. 2.2). It has been predicted that the annual total of lung cancer deaths among women actually will surpass those among men by about the year 2000.

Three

ENUMERATION

When you can measure what you are speaking about,
and express it in numbers, you know something about
it; but when you cannot measure it, when you cannot
express it in numbers, your knowledge is of a meager
and unsatisfactory kind.

—William Thompson, Lord Kelvin
(1824–1907)

DEALING WITH NUMBERS

A coin is flipped 100 consecutive times and the results noted. At each toss, the probability is 50 percent that the coin will turn up heads. Does this mean that it will turn up heads 50 times out of the 100 tosses? No. Why not? We should try to visualize the 100 tosses as constituting only a small random sample out of the entire unknown "universe" of all coin tosses that will (or even can) ever be made. In theory, the coin will indeed have turned up heads in half of the almost infinite number of tosses in this "universe," but a sample of 100 tosses is minuscule by comparison and will show the variations inherent in small samples. If the coin turned up heads 60 times, tails 40 times, is the coin unbalanced? Not necessarily; we can calculate that a ratio of 60 to 40 will occur by pure random chance in about 12 percent of such samples of 100, or in 1 sample out of 8. A ratio of 67 to 33, approximately 2 to 1, can occur by chance in 1.67 percent of samples, or in roughly 1 sample out of 60; and even a ratio of 75 to 25, 3 to 1, can occur by random chance in about $\frac{1}{60}$ of 1 percent, or 1 out of 6,000 samples of 100 tosses apiece.

Living creatures of the same species differ from each other in every possible way, not just in simple yes-or-no, black-or-white, heads-or-tails differences, but in subtle variations such as resistance to disease, longevity, ability to tolerate injury, or ability to respond to a treatment. Faced with questions of the validity of differences between population samples that are being compared, such as between an experimental group and a control group, biologic science calculates the probability that a measured difference between the groups may be due simply to variations in sampling. By convention, differences are regarded as "significant" when the probability that they are due only to sampling error is less than 5 percent, or 1 chance out of 20 (written as $P < 0.05$). Underlying all tests of significance is the "null hypothesis," the assumption that there is no valid difference between the groups; but the null hypothesis is rejected as unlikely if such probability can be calculated as less than 0.05. Degrees of significance can be very high, as when the value of P is less than 0.001, or 1 chance in 1,000. In this case the presumption that the groups really are different will be much more secure. Conversely, the null hypothesis cannot be rejected if the value of P is greater than 0.05. At the level of $P = 0.20$, for example, there is 1 chance out of 5 that the observed differences are due solely to sampling error, and we cannot say that the groups differ from each other.

Suppose that a new chemotherapeutic agent ("Drug A") with possible activity against cancer is being given its first clinical trial. At several cooperating medical centers, sixty consecutive patients with recurrent, inoperable colo-rectal cancer and approximately the same level of performance status agree to enter the trial. Thirty-one are randomly assigned to receive Drug A, twenty-nine to receive an inactive agent, or placebo, as a control group. Drug A and the placebo are distributed to cooperating institutions in coded preparations so that neither the patients nor physicians know which is being administered. The first comparison of survival between groups is made at one year after start of treatment. At this point, twelve patients are surviving out of thirty-one who received Drug A (38.7 percent), while seven of twenty-nine who received the inactive agent are surviving (24.1 percent). The test was designed to answer the question, "Does this new drug increase survival rates at one year in patients with inoperable colo-rectal cancer and good performance status?" The casual observer would say that the answer is obvious; treatment with Drug A was associated with higher survival at one year, compared to the control group. The probability that this difference is due to sampling error, however, can be calculated as slightly over 30 percent, written as $P > 0.3$. The null hypothesis cannot be rejected, and the clinical trial has produced no reliable evidence that Drug A is able to prolong survival in this class of patients.

STUDIES OF SMOKING AND LUNG CANCER

The paper by Wynder and Graham in 1950 found that the great majority of patients with lung cancer had been long-time heavy smokers; few nonsmokers had developed the disease. It was a finding of guilt by past association, retrospective in character, and still objectionable to some analysts as proof of cause. More convincing would be "prospective" studies; those, for example, that initially enrolled a considerable segment of the population, and over a number of years recorded all major illnesses, deaths, and the causes of death within the group. The ideal study would follow all enrolled persons until death, but unfortunately this is seldom practical. Also, our population is mobile, so that many persons will have moved during the study period and will have to be traced. After sufficient time has passed for attrition to have taken place in all groups, calculations can be made to establish the significance of such factors as cigarette consumption per day, years of smoking, and the like, to the probability of development of lung cancer.

Physicians themselves would be an ideal study group, if their cooperation could be secured on a large scale. In 1951 the British Medical Association sent a detailed questionnaire on smoking habits to all its members, with an invitation to participate in a long-term study. (The smoking habit was prevalent even among physicians at that time, only a year after the report of Wynder and Graham.) Replies were received from 30,440 men; because the numbers of women physicians were disproportionately small, the study was restricted to the men. Virtually all were followed for over twenty years, and a certified cause was obtained for each of the 10,072 deaths. Britain's two foremost medical statisticians, Dr. Richard Doll and Richard Peto, directed the study and reported its findings in 1976.[1]

Doll and Peto noted, first, that risk of death from lung cancer increased directly with the number of cigarettes smoked per day. Nonsmokers were subject to a minimum irreducible death rate from lung cancer of 11 per 100,000 per year. Among those who smoked from 1 to 14 cigarettes per day, death rate rose to 78 per 100,000 per year; for those who smoked 15 to 24 per day, 127; and for smokers of 25 or more per day, 251 (Fig. 3.1).

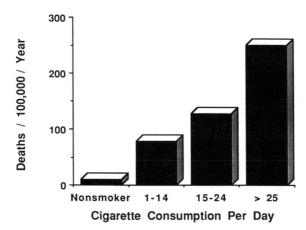

Figure 3.1. Lung cancer mortality rates among male British doctors, by daily cigarette consumption. (Source: Ref. 3–1.)

The association of smoking with development of lung cancer carries a very high degree of significance, $P < 10^{-9}$, or less than one chance in one billion that differences between smokers and nonsmokers were due to sampling.

If cigarette smoking is indeed the cause of lung cancer, quitting should have at least some beneficial effect on the level of risk. All those physicians who had quit smoking, but for less than five years, had a death rate equal to 102 percent of the rate calculated for continuing smokers, essentially identical. Five, however, had quit only after having developed lung cancer. If these five were removed from the analysis, the observed risk for this group dropped to 68 percent of the level for continuing smokers. Comparative risk fell to 35 percent for those who had quit for five to nine years, and to 28 percent after abstinence for ten to fourteen years. Fifteen years or more after quitting, the lung cancer risk had declined to 11 percent of the level for continuing smokers (fig. 3.2).

Calculated another way, the continued risk of lung cancer was expressed as excess mortality over that of nonsmokers; that is, the ratio of observed deaths to the expected number of deaths among lifelong nonsmokers. A nonsmoker would be assigned a relative risk of 1.0. Among continuing smokers, the ratio of excess risk was 15.8; among those having quit for less than five years, 16.0 times the risk for a nonsmoker. Again, omission of the five who already had developed lung cancer reduces this

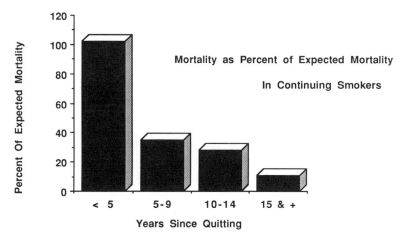

Figure 3.2. Decline in lung cancer death rates after quitting smoking, male British doctors. (Source: Ref. 3–1.)

figure. After five to nine years' abstinence, relative risk had declined to 5.9; after ten to fourteen years to 5.3; and after fifteen years or more to 2.0, twice the risk of a nonsmoker (fig. 3.3).

A study in the United States by Dr. E. Cuyler Hammond found a similar dose-related increase in lung cancer deaths with increasing daily consumption of cigarettes.[2] Men who never had smoked regularly still had a minimum lung cancer death rate of 11.4 per 100,000 per year, identical to that of the nonsmoking male physicians in Great Britain. The death rate increased to 50.2 per 100,000 per year among those who smoked one to nine cigarettes per day, to 89.1 with consumption of ten to nineteen cigarettes per day, and to 151.4 among those who smoked twenty to thirty-nine cigarettes per day. Consumption of forty or more per day resulted in a lung cancer death rate of 205.9 per 100,000 per year (fig. 3.4).

With his associate Dr. Daniel Horn, Hammond found that continued lung cancer risk after quitting varied, depending upon heavy or moderate levels of prior consumption.[3] One cell type, adenocarcinoma, was excluded from the study, since it was believed at the time that lung cancers of this type bore no relation to smoking history. Men who had smoked less than a pack per day, and continued, had a death rate of 57.6 per 100,000 per year; if they had quit for less than a year, a practically identical rate of 56.1. After one to ten years of abstinence, death rate fell to 35.5; and after

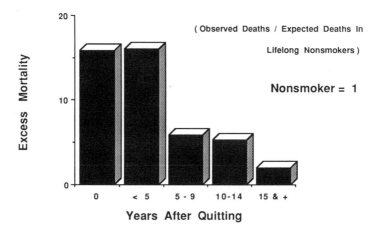

Figure 3.3. Excess continuing lung cancer mortality in ex-smokers, male British doctors. (Source: Ref. 3–1.)

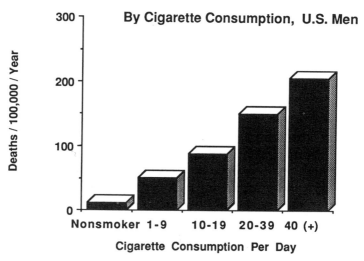

Figure 3.4. Age-standardized lung cancer death rates among U. S. men, by cigarette consumption. (Source: Ref. 3–2.)

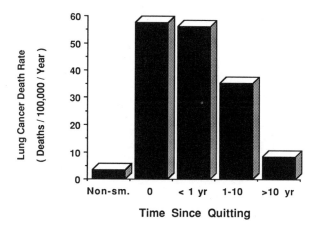

Figure 3.5. Continuing lung cancer death rates, among U. S. male ex-smokers of less than one pack per day. (Source: Ref. 3–3.)

more than ten years, to 8.3, two and a half times the risk level of a nonsmoker (fig. 3.5). Continuing heavy smokers of a pack or more per day, however, had a death rate of 157.1; and if they had quit for less than a year, of 198.0. This seeming paradox reflects a tendency among some smokers to quit only when already in ill health, as did the five British doctors who had quit only after having actually developed lung cancer. Death rate for the heavy smokers after one to ten years of abstinence averaged 77.6, and after more than ten years, 60.5. Sadly, the risk of death from lung cancer among former heavy smokers never declines to the risk level of a lifelong nonsmoker (fig. 3.6).

SECONDHAND SMOKE

The risk of lung cancer resulting from involuntary, or secondhand, smoke exposure is more difficult to define. Careful analysis would have to combine measurement of inhaled smoke concentration times duration of exposure. Houses and workplaces may be ventilated or closed in; non-smoking persons may remain exposed only momentarily or for hours at a time, and from few to many days per month. Just as even a low daily consumption of cigarettes increases the risk of lung cancer, significant and prolonged involuntary smoke exposure does also. A recent study examined lung cancer incidence among nonsmoking wives whose husbands

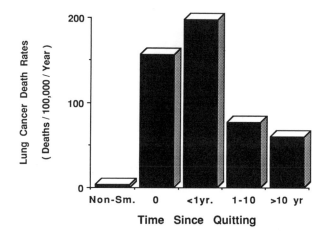

Figure 3.6.. Continuing lung cancer death rates among male ex-smokers of more than one pack per day. (Source: Ref. 3–3.)

smoked twenty or more cigarettes per day.[4] Relative risk of cancer in this group was 2.11; that is, 2.11 times as many women in the study group developed lung cancer as did nonsmoking women not so exposed. Ninety-five percent probability that this difference is not due to sampling error lies within the limits of 1.13 to 3.95 times the nonsmoker's risk; thus we can say that there is less than one chance in twenty that involuntary exposure of this degree did not increase the risk. Another population-based study found a similar twofold increase in the risk of lung cancer among spouses who had never smoked, but who were exposed to smoke at home.[5]

"LOW-YIELD" CIGARETTES

Since the Federal Trade Commission (FTC) began testing cigarettes for tar and nicotine content, manufacturers have outdone each other with claims of lower test levels and safer products. But are "low-yield" cigarettes any safer? A careful study published in 1983 concluded that they are not.[6] The authors compared nicotine content values obtained by FTC testing to those obtained by chemical analysis of the tobacco. FTC testing is done by a machine. A lighted cigarette is placed into a socket, after which a syringe draws a puff of thirty-five milliliters of air through the cigarette once a minute until a specified length of the cigarette has been burned. Nicotine is measured from the puffs of smoke drawn through. The fallacy is that actual nicotine levels in the tobacco do not determine the test results; instead, results are determined by the characteristics of ventilation and of burning. If the cigarette paper is made more porous for the test, a standard drag will pull in more air through the paper, less smoke from the burning end, and test data will say that tar and nicotine levels are very low. This is not simply theory; it is done all the time by manufacturers.

Chemical analysis of the tobacco in cigarettes showed that nicotine content of given brands actually tended to be the reverse of the FTC figures ($P < 0.05$). Levels of a nicotine derivative in smokers' blood samples correlated with the number of cigarettes smoked per day, but did not correlate with the nicotine yield measured by smoking instruments. There is relatively little difference between brands, the study concluded: "Low-yield" cigarettes offer no safety; and, in any case, confirmed smokers will consume enough cigarettes of whatever type to maintain their accustomed nicotine intake.

For the most part, chemicals in the tar condensing from tobacco smoke are the agents that actually cause cancer. If these tars are painted onto a mouse's skin over a period of time, skin cancers form at the site. Nicotine has been regarded as the addicting substance, not necessarily a factor in the development of cancer, but this may be only partially true. Nicotine is a chemical precursor of the compound N-nitroso-nor-nicotine which is strongly carcinogenic in animals, and there are numerous other tobacco-specific N-nitrosamines that are similarly hazardous. Another study found that the risk of myocardial infarction, or heart attack, increased with the number of cigarettes smoked per day, but the risk did not differ between smokers of so-called low-yield and high-yield brands.[7]

RELIGIOUS OR ETHICAL PROHIBITION OF SMOKING

Certain religious groups in the United States discourage or proscribe the use of cigarettes, among them the Church of Jesus Christ of Latter-Day Saints (the Mormons), the Seventh-Day Adventists, and the Old Order Amish. These communities tend to be well-defined and somewhat distinct from the rest of society. The Mormon Church in particular maintains complete and accurate records of its members and their genealogy, and has cooperated in a number of studies. Within the church, use of alcohol, tobacco, coffee, tea, or nonmedicinal drugs is prohibited by the "Word of Wisdom," rules of health given to his followers by Joseph Smith in 1833.[8]

One study found that incidence of smoking-related cancers—those of lung, mouth, tongue, larynx, esophagus, and bladder—was reduced by half among Mormons in Utah as compared to non-Mormons, whatever their smoking habits.[9] Another, even more striking, found that death rates from all cancers combined among observing Mormon males in California and Utah was only half the 1970 cancer death rate among white males in the United States generally.[10] Lung cancer mortality had to be reduced by more than half to achieve this difference.

OTHER CAUSES OF LUNG CANCER

What of the 10 to perhaps 15 percent of lung cancer patients who have not smoked? Another environmental factor has been known since the nineteenth century as a cause of lung cancer; affecting only a few people, this factor had a name and was feared long before cigarette smoking had become widely prevalent. A mountain range in central Europe known as the Erzgebirge, or Ore Mountains, separates the German province of Saxony from the Czechoslovakian province of Bohemia. The "ores" contain the uranium series of naturally radioactive elements. Pitchblende was mined here for Marie and Pierre Curie's laboratory. Virtually all miners who had worked underground for more than five years were known to have died of the "Bergkrankheit" or mountain sickness; eventually this was proved to be lung cancer, of a highly malignant type in most cases.

Uranium and cobalt remain the foremost products of the mines today; unfortunately such ores are of immense strategic importance in the atomic age. The Erzgebirge have been a closed and tightly guarded preserve for many years. At first, the area of the mines spanned the border between Imperial Germany and Austria-Hungary; after the Treaty of Versailles, the border between Germany and Czechoslovakia. Following the Munich agreement of 1938 the area came entirely under the control of Hitler, and after World War II it passed into the possession of the German Democratic Republic and the Peoples' Republic of Czechoslovakia. As a result, the mines lie entirely behind the Iron Curtain.

Early studies of the miners' cancer centered especially in the towns of Schneeberg in Saxony and Joachimsthal in Bohemia; the latter is now renamed Jáchymov. Because of exclusion of Westerners from this area, the last report in an English-language journal may have been the review by Lorenz in 1944.[11] The disease plays no ideological favorites, since lung cancer is an occupational hazard to uranium miners in the western United States,[12] and in other countries as well.[13] There are various indications that the miners' cancer remains a health problem in Central Europe.[14]

Radon inhalation is the cause of miners' lung cancer, possibly of some nonminers' cancers as well. Radon 222 is a colorless, odorless heavy gas, the fourth new element produced by the radioactive decay series beginning with uranium 238. Radon itself is the only gaseous element in this sequence, with a half-life of 3.8 days; in its turn, it decays into a series of short-lived solid elements known collectively as radon daughters, whose half-lives range from fractions of a second to minutes. As a gas, radon can seep from rock strata into the atmosphere in mines or even in the basements of homes, and if decaying after inhalation, deposits its solid radioactive daughters in the lungs. Continued decay of these short-lived daughter elements can subject the lung to cancer-causing doses of radiation; the effect is multiplied by smoking.

Concern has risen in recent years that homes overlying uranium-bearing rock formations may accumulate radon levels hazardous to the occupants, but unfortunately radon levels in room air are unpredictable. Some surveys in the United States have found variations of a hundredfold or greater in levels between private homes, while the highest and lowest levels measured in Canada and in Ireland were found in identical houses standing side by side.[15] The true risk to people in their homes is only poorly understood, but it is clear that in susceptible geographic areas, differences such as ventilation or tightness of homes can affect interior radon levels. Energy-efficient homes may pose a greater hazard to occupants than do loosely-built houses. Estimates of the number of new lung cancer cases caused by radon exposure range from about a thousand to several thousand per year; it is clear that we do not have precise information. By comparison, it is predicted that 155,000 new cases of lung cancer will appear in the U.S. in 1989, and about 142,000 of the patients will die of the disease.[16]

Other possible causes of lung cancer are even less well-defined. Inhalation of certain types of asbestos fibers increases the risk both of lung cancer and of mesothelioma, a malignancy of the pleural surfaces on the outside of the lung.[17] Concurrent smoking multiplies the risk of lung cancer among persons with asbestos exposure, over the risk of either factor alone. An increase in lung cancer incidence was noted especially among shipyard workers exposed to asbestos during World War II.

Nickel and chromate miners are subject to higher risk, again potentiated by smoking.

In our society, cigarette smoking is by far the prime and foremost cause of lung cancer. Few of us are either uranium miners or shipyard workers. All of the statistical reviews indicate that 85 to 90 percent of the people who die of lung cancer would not have died if they had not smoked. The tobacco industry may contend that " *No one* knows what causes cancer" and portray smoking as healthful and pleasurable; but it is not so.

LUNG CANCER AROUND THE WORLD

Death rates from lung cancer vary widely between nations and cultures around the world, the United States not having the highest rates by any means (fig. 3.7). The advanced and developed nations generally have high rates. Scotland has the highest of all. Death rates often are lower in Third World countries but not necessarily; those in the Asian island nation of Singapore actually are slightly higher than those in the United States.[18] The Muslim religion is not necessarily a bar to smoking habits or lung cancer risk in today's world.[19] Per capita cigarette consumption in selected countries around the world is shown graphically in figure 3.8. Cigarette manufacturers see the Third World countries as an enormous potential bonanza because of their vast populations.[20] The more ad-

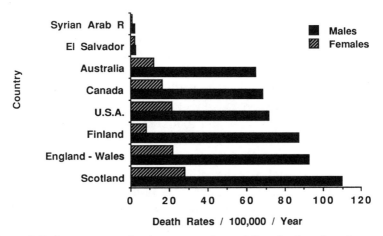

Figure 3.7. Lung cancer death rates, male and female, in selected countries around the world, 1980–1981. (Source: Ref. 3–25.)

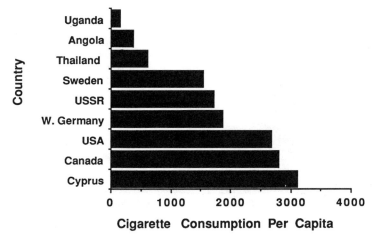

Figure 3.8. Per capita cigarette consumption, in selected countries around the world. (Source: U. S. Department of Agriculture.)

vanced of non-Western countries seem to have adopted the smoking habit even more enthusiastically than the nations of the West. In Japan, one survey found 63 percent of adult males to be smokers, and in at least some provinces of mainland China, a staggering 90 percent.[21] In the poorer nations, craving for cigarettes does not depend in any way upon wealth or affluence, as Bill Hunter had seen among the poverty-stricken German civilians after World War II.

MARIJUANA VERSUS TOBACCO

Is marijuana less of a risk factor for lung cancer because it is not tobacco? A comparative study of smoking of the two agents suggests that it is definitely more of a risk.[22] Smoking of marijuana was associated with at least a threefold increase in the amount of tar inhaled, and with retention in the respiratory tract of one-third more inhaled tar (P < 0.001). While smoking marijuana, the subjects took larger puffs, inhaled more deeply, and held an inhaled breath longer than they did while smoking tobacco. These smoking dynamics and the delivery of tar during marijuana smoking were only slightly influenced by content of the active alkaloid, delta-9-tetra-hydro-cannabinol. Were these effects a factor in Andrew Cunningham's cancer at a young age? Possibly; but one case proves nothing, and it is likely that Andrew also had some factors of individual susceptibility.

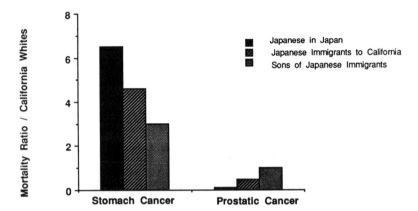

Figure 3.9. Changes in cancer incidence at two sites, among Japanese immigrants to California. (Source: Ref. 3–25.)

GENETIC PREDISPOSITION AND THE QUESTION OF MICRO-NUTRIENTS

Clearly, not every person will develop lung cancer after the same duration and intensity of exposure to cigarette smoke; this uncertainty points to variations in individual susceptibility, primarily genetic in origin. To date we have little knowledge of the precise factors, or any control over them; but genes have been identified that apparently predispose individuals to development of certain types of lung cancer.[23]

Hitherto unknown dietary or environmental factors may possibly be important in the development of cancer. Incidence rates of certain cancers differ greatly between countries and may change following emigration from the homeland to another country. Considerable study has been given to populations of Japanese immigrants in California and their children.[24] Stomach cancer is prevalent in Japan, for example, and cancer of the prostate relatively rare; but the rates among immigrants and their children change progressively toward those prevalent among whites in California (fig. 3.9). In other studies, a high fiber content in the diet is clearly related to a lower incidence of colo-rectal cancer. Much interest has arisen in the possibility that changes in trace dietary factors may either favor or inhibit the development of certain cancers, independent of the factor of smoking.

Retinoids (Vitamin A and its synthetic analogues) and some of the vitamin A precursors (principally beta-carotene) have come under the closest scrutiny. These compounds have inhibitory effects on development of cancer in small laboratory animals; it appears that they are capable of controlling cell growth rates, thereby favoring cell differentiation in various epithelial tissues. The carotenoids may be capable also of minimizing tissue and chromosome damage by free-oxygen radicals, a potentially protective action. At present these effects remain at least partially hypothetical. In human cancer, lung cancer in particular, some retrospective studies have suggested a beneficial effect,[25] while others have failed to show any benefit.[26] For the time being, the evidence remains inconclusive, but prospective clinical trials are under way that should eventually provide clear evidence for or against a protective effect by these compounds.

Four

SOME YOUNG PATIENTS

But if my case bee as Saint *Paules* case, *quotidie morior,* that I *die dayly,* that something heavier than death falls upon me every day; If my case be *Davids* case, *tota die mortificamur; all the day long wee are killed,* that not onely every day, but every houre of the day some thing heavier than death falls upon me, . . Yet *Domini Domini sunt exitus mortis,* with God *the Lord* are the issues of death.

—John Donne, *Death's Duell* (last Sermon,
February 25, 1630)

ELAINE SCHMIDT. NOVEMBER 1977.

Elaine Schmidt had been coughing all night, unable to stop, and she felt worn out in the morning. This had gone on for more than a month, and was getting worse. She had no personal physician; a week previously, feeling feverish, she had gone to the emergency room at St. Luke's Hospital. The doctor had obtained blood counts and a chest X-ray, told her that the film showed a shadow in the right lung, probably representing pneumonia, and had let her go home with a prescription for an antibiotic. The fever and sputum had declined somewhat, but her cough had persisted. This morning, feeling worse, she asked her neighbor to look in on the two children and called a taxicab to take her back to St. Luke's.

Seeing her exhaustion, the doctor in the emergency room advised that she be admitted to the hospital. The staff physician taking medical admissions that day was Dr. Ted Thompson. Elaine called her mother, and asked her to pick up the children. After she had been admitted, and settled in a room, Dr. Thompson came in to meet her and to review her entire problem.

Elaine was thirty-three; she had been born in Springfield, Massachusetts, but her parents were retired now in Taunton. She had been married at twenty-one, had two children now aged ten and seven. She and her husband were separated, and he was living in New Jersey. She had been doing clerical work for the New Bedford National Bank, had quit work at the beginning of the summer to look after the children, but the bank had had no place available for her when school reopened in September. Elaine had undergone an appendectomy at age eighteen and biopsy of a lump in her breast (benign) at age twenty-five. Otherwise she had been in fairly good health. She had begun smoking at age seventeen, smoked about a pack per day since then. Her paternal grandfather had died of lung cancer, as had a paternal uncle, at the age of forty-two. Elaine had lost about ten pounds since her symptoms had begun. Dr. Thompson noted her racking cough, made worse by talking, and heard a slight change in the breath sounds over the lower portion of her right lung. She was thin and appeared exhausted. He noted no other obvious abnormalities during his examination. He left orders that she should receive a mild sedative when necessary, also frequent doses of a codeine cough syrup, and specified that all sputum, any phlegm she could raise, be sent for culture. For the time being he did not seriously consider lung cancer as a cause of her problem; she was young, and tuberculosis or some similar infection seemed more likely.

Subsequent chest X-rays continued to show a poorly defined density in the area of the right hilum, the "root" of the right lung. Microscopic examination and cultures of her sputum failed to identify any pathogenic or disease-causing bacteria, and stained smears persistently failed to reveal the acid-fast bacilli characteristic of tuberculosis. A skin test for TB was negative. The racking cough continued in spite of medication. After a few days, with no good answers available, Dr. Thompson decided to have her transferred to one of the large hospitals in Boston.

Her physician at the new hospital found her hoarse, exhausted by coughing. New X-rays of her chest showed no clearing of the density in the lung. He asked for consultation from a thoracic surgeon, to do bronchoscopy and mediastinoscopy, examination of the interior of the bronchial tubes plus a surgical biopsy of the lymph nodes within the middle partition of the chest. He and the surgeon agreed that the procedure would be tolerable for Elaine only if she were given a general anesthetic. The surgeon could see narrowing of the bronchial passageway to the middle and lower lobes on the right; he took biopsies which later revealed undifferentiated or anaplastic carcinoma, one of the variants of lung cancer. Enlarged lymph nodes were found in the mediastinum and biopsies taken from the uppermost two or three, but these failed to show involvement by the cancer. Scans of the possible sites of tumor spread—brain, liver, and bones—proved grossly normal. Elaine's physician sat down with her for a serious talk and mentioned first that the diagnosis of lung cancer now was clear. She was angry and sad over the news but after a day or two was more reconciled to it. Surgical removal of the lung appeared to be the key to possible treatment; so far, no absolute contraindication had appeared. The cough was wearing her out and only removal of the tumor promised any chance of relief. Removal of the entire lung would be necessary. Elaine was still upset and at first demurred, but the next day changed her mind and agreed to the surgery.

At the operation, the surgeon found the large tumor mass close in the hilum, the "root" of the lung. Lymph nodes around the hilum were swollen and hardened by tumor involvement; similar nodes extended into the mediastinum. To his dismay, the surgeon could see that the nodes he had previously biopsied and found to be clear of tumor lay just above those that were obviously involved. This degree of spreading practically eliminated any chance of cure by surgical removal, but the pain and disability resulting from the operation already were unavoidable. The surgeon removed the lung with the aim of at least relieving her intractable cough.

Elaine's recovery was slow. Although her cough was improved, she was depressed and weakened by the pain. She received doses of morphine at frequent intervals; in addition, intercostal nerve blocks were done three times during the couple of days that she was in the intensive care unit. The nurses first helped her out of bed into a chair on the day after the operation, and began walking her with assistance on the second day. She remained disabled by the pain, seemingly out of proportion to most patients' reaction to comparable surgery. She was hardly willing to move or to do anything by herself. In spite of her young age, she could not be discharged from the hospital until the thirteenth day.

A consultation with the radiotherapists had been arranged before her discharge, aiming to treat the involved nodes in the mediastinum. She plainly needed more time for recovery; treatment was not started until two weeks after her discharge and continued on weekdays for three more weeks.

From that time on, her existence was a constant strain. She was unable to look after the children following her return home, and could only depend on her parents to help. There was a readmission to St. Luke's Hospital when her pain could no longer be controlled at home; her physician sought to change and readjust the medication schedules. She never was able to eat well and could not recover her strength. Months later, there were new pains in her right shoulder and in several ribs; a bone scan and new X-rays indicated that the tumor had spread to these bones. Chemotherapy was offered to her, but without much promise of benefit, and she had several brief hospital admissions to receive it. Subsequently she was admitted a final time, near death, and expired about thirteen months after the first diagnosis of her cancer.

DR. BILL HUNTER. OCTOBER 1981.

Bill Hunter's older son, Clark, had entered medical school in New York City this fall. At the end of August, Bill and his wife had rented a station wagon for the weekend to move him there. Clark previously had attended a small, selective liberal arts college in upstate New York. He loved the school and enjoyed his entire time there, graduating with high honors and election to Phi Beta Kappa. Most of his applications to medical schools had brought invitations to interview; a number had brought offers of acceptance, but he had wished to attend school away from home. New York City had always held a strong attraction for him. Fortunately the school he chose maintained two student dormitories; the quarters for first-year students resembled cubicles in a monastery, but at least they provided available and convenient housing in mid-Manhattan at a price not beyond reason. The upperclass students' dormitory around the corner on Seventieth Street promised improved comforts and amenities for survivors of the freshman year.

This year, for the first time, the medical college had planned a parents' weekend for the first year class. There was to be no football game as there had been at the colleges, but instead a program on Friday afternoon devoted to problems in medical education, the students' transition from college, and the special features of the school and medical center by the East River. The remainder of the weekend was to be kept free. Bill and his wife took the train down to New York for the sake of a leisurely trip and stayed at their favorite small hotel near the Metropolitan Museum of Art. They met Clark for lunch on Friday, then went to the afternoon session while Clark returned to classes. The parents' meeting opened with a welcome by the dean of the medical college; he discussed the aims and special concerns of the school for about ten minutes. Other professors spoke briefly, upper-class students described the school and the New York experience, and a student quartet sang three selections. The next speaker was introduced as a professor of medicine whose special concern was with human values in medicine. Bill's attention was caught suddenly when the speaker asked whether compassion and concern for sick people could be taught to students, or otherwise ingrained if at least some students did not already possess them. "Why not?" the speaker asked. "We think nothing of teaching them, verbatim, the entire chemical pathway of anaerobic glycolysis. Does it follow that we can't teach personal sensitivity to a sick person's needs and fears?" With only a few minutes allotted to him, the speaker went on to point out that relief of the patient's fear and suffering must be the physician's ultimate concern. Suffering is equated in most people's minds with pain, but wrongly, and few physicians have considered the distinction or even are aware of it. Too often, in this oversight the medical profession had missed its calling and its greatest opportunity.

Bill was startled by the speaker's discussion, together with others in the audience, and forced to concede to himself that never before had he confronted this critical distinction, nor understood its implications. In his formative years, no teacher had challenged him to think in these terms. "Pain and suffering"—that was the phrase beloved by all the lawyers seeking damages for their injured clients. It was simple; a person in pain was suffering, and the phrase had become fixed in common usage. Were the two concepts really so different as the speaker had said? The question kept coming back to him, long after the weekend was over.

A few months later, in March, Bill found an extended discussion of the problem of suffering, by the speaker at the weekend session in New York, in one of the medical journals. This time the author expanded his thesis considerably, but again he emphasized the difference: pain is experienced by the body, suffering by the whole person. Pain and suffering often are associated, but either can exist without the other. In simplest terms, suffering is the torment of being deprived of control over the future, the loss of hope that life may again be set right. It originates from adversity threatening destruction of the person, or of the person's ability to function in his or her perceived role. We have got to do away, he said, with the Cartesian distinction between body on the one hand and "person" or "mind" on the other; unfortunately medicine has concerned itself with the former, and in the present day often disregards hurts that afflict the person. It does not follow that physicians always are able to relieve suffering, or even to prevent it. Often, they may not be able to redress or undo the catastrophic destruction of a life's prospects. But if they fail to understand the loss and anguish at the root of a patient's suffering, physicians unwittingly may be responsible for its cause, or more often for its continuation.[1] Some patients are able to overcome their suffering and regain wholeness and integrity in spite of pain and the prospect of death, through resort to the transcendent dimension that makes up a part of their character and belief. This characteristic is deeply personal, differing from one individual to another.

ANDREW CUNNINGHAM. OCTOBER 1982.

Andy tossed his books into the knapsack, went outside to his old Chevy, and drove to the campus for another day of classes. He was a sophomore this year, not particularly fond of college but going out of a sense that years were passing without enough accomplishment on his part, or with good enough prospects for his future. At twenty-six, he was older than his classmates and he couldn't get involved with many of their enthusiasms.

Andy had enlisted in the army after high school; fortunately the Vietnam War had long since been over and his tour was neither rigorous nor dangerous. He felt no attraction to a career in the army, but his service time had accumulated credits toward college tuition, making it easier for him to be here. Otherwise, the army had done him no favors. Midway through the hitch, boredom and peer pressure had started him smoking marijuana, and he remained an avid frequent user more than four years later. In between, he smoked ordinary cigarettes, but while doing so he still craved the grass. After discharge, he had supported himself by various odd jobs until he could enroll, much to his parents' relief, at Fitchburg State College. It was an advantage for him to live at home and drive to classes.

This morning his knees and ankles were painful as he walked. There had been some stiffness and a few twinges of pain during the last week or two, but he had thought nothing of them. He had felt tired recently, almost worn out at the end of the day. He did not bother watching his weight; with a tall, lanky build, weight had never been of any concern to him. But all day the soreness nagged at him, and in subsequent days it grew more severe to the point where walking was a strain. Looking at his ankles in the evening, he was startled to see them swollen, painful to pressure, the skin somewhat thickened and discolored over them. Also, his fingers looked oddly different from what he remembered, now somewhat bulbous in shape at the tips, with the nails curved in a longitudinal direction. On hearing all this, his mother insisted that she take him to see the family's doctor the next day.

Dr. Terence Carney was puzzled by the oddity of Andy's complaint, especially since there had been no injury or severe exertion. Andy's ankle joints were plainly inflamed, the knees also but less so, but the symmetrical pattern looked unusual. His difficulties should respond to one of the anti-inflammatory drugs plus a few days' rest, Dr. Carney was sure. He gave Andy a prescription for ibuprofen tablets and an appointment to return in two weeks.

Andy's pain and soreness were considerably relieved for several weeks, but the swelling and discoloration of his ankles did not go away. He returned to his studies, only moderately limited for ordinary daily activities. After two months, in spite of the medication, the pain and disability again grew worse. Now there was also a constant pain, dull at first but becoming more severe, which seemed to be located in the lower rib cage on the left side of his chest. This time Dr. Carney had him admitted to Leominster Hospital for a serious evaluation. In the hospital he had intermittent low-grade fever. The red-cell sedimentation rate was elevated and serum levels of a bone enzyme, alkaline phosphatase, were elevated as well. All these were consistent with some form of arthritis; there was no answer so far. X-ray films of his wrists, knees, and ankles showed no fractures or displacements; but there was a thin layering of new bone over the normal bony contours near these joints. Chest X-rays showed only some streaky markings in the lower lobe of the left lung, a nonspecific pattern with no certain significance, while a computerized tomographic, or CT, scan confirmed the streaky pattern but also indicated the presence of a small amount of fluid in the chest cavity nearby, just outside the lung. A bone scan after injection of a small dose of a radioactive tracer compound showed a pattern of increased bone turnover activity, appearing as "hot areas," in the long bones adjacent to his knees, ankles, wrists, and even knuckles. Once more, the distribution of these hot areas was completely symmetrical between right and left sides. Scanning of the lungs with another isotope tracer showed marked disparity between blood flow and air ventilation in the left lower lobe. The nuclear medicine consultant suggested that this pattern might represent pulmonary embolus, the lodging of a blood clot in the pulmonary artery. After discussion, he and Dr. Carney agreed that Andy should be transferred without delay to a larger medical center in Boston.

The ambulance ride took only an hour, and Andy was admitted to the John C. Warren Memorial Hospital, overlooking the Back Bay fens. There were numerous additional tests, but his doctors' concern began to focus on the increasing pain in his chest, the seemingly nonspecific streaky markings seen on the X-rays of his lungs, and the adjacent small collection of fluid. An ounce or two of the fluid was obtained by needle tap, and was found on microscopic examination to contain large irregular malignant cells. After suitable sedation, bronchoscopy was performed, again with a slim, flexible fiberoptic scope; no obvious tumor mass was seen but specimens obtained by brushing and saline irrigation from the left lung contained large numbers of malignant cells. Now the parts of the puzzle were beginning to fall into place. The disabling pain, swelling, and tenderness in knees and ankles, with the bulbous enlargement or "clubbing" of his fingertips, together make up a rare but distinctive warning sign in a few cases of lung cancer. The combination is known by an awkward name, hypertrophic pulmonary osteoarthropathy. Translated into everyday English, it would be "enlarging affliction of bones and joints, related to the lung." In abbreviated medical terminology, it often is referred to as HPOA or even more simply as OA, osteoarthropathy. How the cancer occasionally produces this warning sign in the joints is unknown; it is known, however, that successful clean surgical removal of the lung tumor often is followed by immediate disappearance of the bone and joint pains. For all the possibility of dramatic relief, the long-term outlook for such patients is poor and the chances of a cancer cure are slight. The astonishing paradox in Andy's case was that lung cancer should have appeared in one so young, but it had been reported to occur, however rarely, in children and even in infants.

In the hospital, Andy complained of rapidly increasing pain in the left side of his chest. Soon he was pleading and begging for more narcotics long before his next doses were due. To the resident staff at the Warren Memorial, looking after his daily needs, it appeared that Andy had an abnormally low threshold for pain. Was it related to his heavy indulgence in marijuana for the last several years? By only the fourth or fifth evening after his admission, each dose of morphine would hold his pain in abeyance for barely more than an hour; then he would become more and more agitated, sometimes writhing and sobbing. Distressed and bewildered by the apparent severity of his pain, but feeling obliged to do something about it, the young house doctor allowed him doses at his own request, after any period of more than an hour. Thereafter, Andy often appeared somewhat lethargic, but for the moment, content. The young residents had no stomach to resist or deny his continuous demands for more morphine. If the pain were real it must be intolerable, and the frequent doses continued.

How could his cancer be treated effectively? With this particular cell type of lung cancer, the only possibility of cure lies in a completely successful surgical removal. Complete removal was out of the question—impossible because first, cancer cells had been found in the pleural fluid collection, outside the lung. Also, the distribution and severity of his pain meant that the tumor must be invading a large area of the chest wall, outside the lung. A consultant from the Radiation Therapy Department expressed his dismay at the apparent severity of Andy's pain. He advised that in his opinion, effective relief of the pain could not be obtained from radiation treatment alone. Almost the entire left side of the chest wall appeared to be involved; all of this large area would have to be irradiated to a high dose level; there would be destructive effects on the lung in particular, while the chance of significant relief of his pain would be slight. Other consultants, medical oncologists from the Lowell-Eliot Cancer Institute, saw him for consideration of treatment by chemotherapy. The tumor cell type, once more, was unfavorable; few if any such tumors ever showed a significant response. The oncologists from the cancer institute agreed, however, to accept responsibility for his care while any and all possible avenues for treatment were explored. His narcotic consumption remained a problem. Assuming that any effective treatment plan could be worked out, there seemed less reason for it if he were to be hopelessly addicted afterward.

In this impasse, there were no easy or particularly hopeful solutions. The oncologists decided to begin by consultation with a thoracic surgeon. Was it possible that his OA, the osteoarthropathy, might be at least partially relieved if the lung could be removed? Also, might radiation treatment of his chest wall be more feasible or effective if the lung were no longer in the way to be injured? Dr. Bill Hunter was asked to review the problem and consider surgical removal even if incomplete, the other possible treatments to be left until afterward. To Bill, Andy's prospects looked grim and dismal, but doctors no less than others are sometimes swayed by the argument, "We have to do something; we can't leave the patient like this." With an uneasy sense that it was contrary to his better judgment, he discussed the operation with Andy and his parents. They were prepared to consider whatever was advised. Bill was plainly worried that Andy's heavy use of narcotics would make it almost impossible to look after him properly. He would need to have Andy awake and reasonably cooperative following the operation, able to do the coughing, clearing out the remaining lung, begin getting out of bed, and all the other things necessary to his recovery.

At the operation, a poorly defined mass density was found within the lung, representing the primary tumor; also there were numerous implants of tumor tissue on the surface of the lung itself and on the inside surface of the chest wall. The lung was removed without particular difficulty, but there was no way of effectively removing all the remaining implants. With the aim of controlling his pain, three intercostal nerves above the incision and five below it were identified as they emerged from the spinal column, one running just below each rib. The individual nerve trunks were frozen twice in succession with a special probe chilled by liquid nitrogen, a procedure called cryoablation. In addition, after the operation had been completed, a tiny plastic catheter was placed by the anesthesiologist into the epidural space just outside the spinal cord and its coverings, for injection of small repeated doses of medication to control the pain later on.

Andy was young and tolerated the massive surgical procedure itself without difficulty. During his recovery period depression, pain, disability, and the effects of his increasing doses of narcotics combined to make him almost helpless. Soon it was impossible to say whether he had received any benefit at all from the operation. Radiation treatments were begun as soon as he was out of bed, and eventually he was released from the hospital with what was thought to be liberal provision of narcotics, to be taken as needed for the pain.

Andy was out of the hospital a little more than a week. His complaints of increasing disability and unbearable pain brought about readmission, and soon he was again getting the morphine doses almost hourly. It appeared necessary to discontinue the radiation treatments; after two weeks of treatment, he insisted that the pain was only getting worse. There were more consultations, this time with neurosurgeons in the hope that one of the newer approaches to pain relief might be possible; but the consultants declined to consider major or destructive surgical procedures because of his advanced disease. A schedule of medications was set up in a different way; every six hours he received a large dose of a long-acting narcotic, methadone, with doses of tranquilizing drugs between times together with additional doses of ordinary morphine when needed. On this program he was again released from the hospital. There could be no thought any more of further treatment of his cancer; Andy's condition had deteriorated to the point at which nothing mattered but the relief of his pain.

At home he lay around most of the time, ate poorly or not at all, made no efforts to increase his activity or to begin getting out of the house. Already thin, he continued to lose weight. Narcotic drugs were provided to him liberally; there was no other possible course. Dazed with the medication, he yet continued to suffer because he remained aware of the disintegration of his personal identity. There was one more brief admission to the hospital for supportive care, then finally a readmission because he was rapidly approaching a terminal state. Andy died two days later, less than four months in all after his cancer had first been discovered.

Andrew's illness had manifested itself by severe pain from the first day to the last. If suffering is not necessarily the same thing as pain, we must wonder which troubled him the more. Did his illness also cause him great suffering? Without having good access to his state of mind through those few months, we would have to believe that it did. Why? He had received large quantities of narcotic drugs intended to relieve the pain, and at times was in a relaxed semi-stupor from them. The pain of his illness must have been absent or at any rate suppressed at such times, but his suffering must have become intolerable.

Until the time when he was found to have an incurable malignancy, at the age of only twenty-six, Andy had the prospect of a future stretching ahead of him, which included his education, a career, continued challenge and opportunity. He had a supporting family and a number of friends. His personhood remained intact. His pain at this time was annoying and troublesome, but it did not constitute suffering. When the realization of incurable disease was forced on him, everything changed; no longer did he have any control over his future; even the imminent destruction of his person had become inevitable. Now the intense suffering could no longer be avoided. His pain became unbearable because he no longer had any grounds for hope.

Five

YOUTH IS DIFFERENT

You young debaters over the doctrine
Of the soul's immortality,
I who lie here was the village atheist,
Talkative, contentious, versed in the arguments
Of the infidels.
But through a long sickness
Coughing myself to death
I read the *Upanishads* and the poetry of Jesus.
And they lighted a torch of hope and intuition
And desire which the Shadow,
Leading me swiftly through the caverns of darkness
Could not extinguish.

—Edgar Lee Masters, *Spoon River Anthology*
(1914)

LUNG CANCER IN CHILDREN, A BIOLOGIC ODDITY

Cancer is associated in our minds with middle and older age; the tragic occurrence of cancer in children evokes special sympathy. Much of childhood cancer takes the form of leukemia and the related lymphomas such as Hodgkin's disease, but it may also occur in the bones as osteogenic sarcoma, or in or near the kidneys, especially in infancy. Chemotherapy, by itself or in combination with surgery and radiation, tends to be much more effective against childhood cancers than against the common malignancies of adult life; the reasons are not entirely clear. Cancer death rates among children in the United States have been reduced dramatically since 1950. The death rate from leukemia has been cut by half; that from Hodgkin's disease by 80 percent; that from bone cancer by about half;

and from kidney cancer by 75 percent.[1] Only a few, relatively rare adult cancers can be controlled to anything like the same degree, while the common ones are virtually unresponsive. Death rates from the commonest of all, lung cancer, continue to increase at a rapid rate.

Most cases of lung cancer result from long-continued cigarette smoking, but perhaps 10 to as many as 15 percent occur independently of a smoking history. A few of these have appeared in young people, children, or very rarely even in infants. Clearly these bear no relation to smoking but have to be regarded as randomly occurring biologic oddities for which we have no good explanation. A recent review analyzed forty-seven cases reported since 1876 of lung cancer in children under the age of sixteen. The youngest patient was five months old; nine were less than three years old.[2] All the cell types of lung cancer were represented in this group, but with a notable minority of the common adult squamous-cell carcinoma; 80 percent of the children's cases were adenocarcinoma and undifferentiated carcinoma. The disease process usually was widespread and incurable at the time of diagnosis. Average survival of the forty-seven children was only seven months, and the only cancers probably cured had been discovered in Japan during mass X-ray surveys of school children for tuberculosis. Four of these children were alive and free of disease from three to eight years after surgical removal of the lung.

We must recognize that lung cancer can occur in children and even infants, but these instances are rare, random, or even freakish in distribution, and without known cause. Smoking cannot be the causative factor, as it is in almost all adults. Children have done poorly in spite of treatment, and only a few have been cured.

LUNG CANCER IN YOUNG ADULTS

In adult life, age under forty years is considered "young" in relation to cancer onset. Age forty to fifty is an intermediate level, and cancer occurrence becomes more common beyond the age of fifty. In the distribution by age-groups of those forty and under, but with children excluded, the relation of lung cancer to smoking is more clearly apparent.

Five different studies of the disease in young persons, aged forty and under, have shown remarkable similarity; three were from the United States, one each from Canada and Great Britain.[3] A sixth study[4] examined lung cancer incidence in men in the United States aged forty-five and under. Below the age of thirty, lung cancer remains rare and freakish in

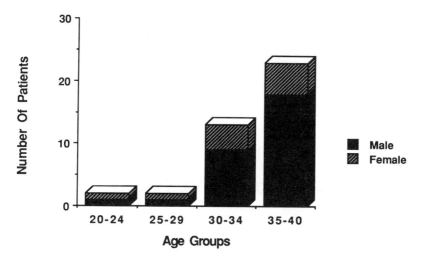

Figure 5.1. Distribution of new lung cancer cases in young adults aged 40 and below in Great Britain, by age-groups and sex. (Source: Ref. 5–3.)

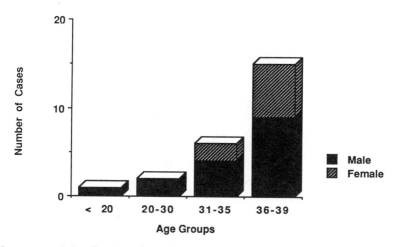

Figure 5.2. Distribution of new lung cancer cases in young adults below age 40 in the United States, by age-groups and sex. (Source: Ref. 5–4.)

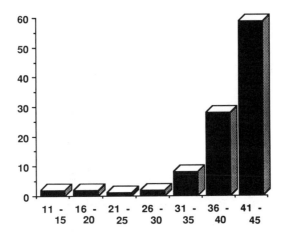

Figure 5.3. Distribution of new cases of lung cancer in young men aged 45 and below in the United States, by age-groups. (Source: Ref. 5–8.)

distribution. The smoking habit often is acquired as early as age twelve to fifteen, as it was by Terry Barton for example, but its effect upon each user is not clearly predictable and varies widely because of individual susceptibility. Most persons do not develop lung cancer until after nearly twenty years of smoking, or more; the usual exposure is distinctly longer.

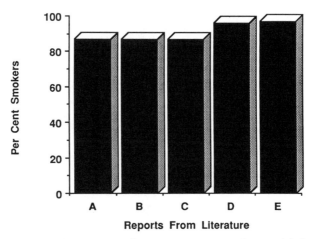

Figure 5.4. Percent cigarette smokers among new patients with lung cancer aged 40 and under: Sum of five reports. (Source: Refs. 5–3 through 5–8.)

A precipitous rise in the number of cases begins after age thirty, more after age thirty-five (figs. 5.1, 5.2, 5.3); both men and women share in this abrupt onset.

I have noted that the disease in childhood bears no association with smoking, but there are only the barest few cases in children. In the five studies of adult patients under age forty,[5] from 87 to 97 percent of the patients were heavy smokers (fig. 5.4). Young age at smoking onset, added to the minimum time lag of close to twenty years, correlates well with the sharp rise in numbers of cases at around age thirty-five. From this age on, the disease retains its close association with the prime causative factor.

Are there any other notable differences in young adult life? Two of the studies listed proportions of cases in which the tumor was strictly localized (that is, not spreading) at the time of removal. One study found that only 8.7 percent of the patients had localized disease,[6] the other found 9.6 percent;[7] identical figures when we remember sampling variation. In older age groups, however, the proportion of cases with localized disease *increases* with each successive decade, reaching 42 percent in patients aged eighty or over.[8] These figures point to a gradual diminution in the malignant behavior of lung cancer with increasing age of the host, since rapid growth and spread are indicators of degree of malignancy. Reasons for the gradual decline are not yet understood. Chances of cure by surgical removal depend heavily on the disease being localized. Even if the degree of malignancy diminishes gradually with increasing age, the host tends to become less able to tolerate the major surgery necessary for treatment.

Six

NATURAL HISTORY OF THE DISEASE

Life is short, the Art long;
The moment fleeting,
Experience fallacious,
And decision difficult.

—Hippocrates (c. 460–400 B.C.)

The man of science has learned to believe in justification, not by faith, but by verification.

—Thomas Henry Huxley (1825–1895).

ORIGIN OF THE MALIGNANT CELL

All tissues are made up of cells—living units of microscopic size, each equipped with the chemical machinery to extract energy from substrates or food compounds, to build proteins that the cell needs for growth, repair, and any specialized functions it may perform; and, up to a point at least, to reproduce itself. This last function requires that each cell possess all the genetic information of the parent organism plus coded instructions for creating the animal and maintaining it in active vigorous life.

If each cell possesses full genetic information, are the cells potentially immortal? Not as they normally exist in our bodies, or even in tissue culture after being taken out of our bodies. Under these conditions the cells age after they differentiate, gradually lose special functions, eventually can no longer reproduce themselves, and die. They have died of old age, so to speak, or else one might say that the controlling program has restricted their indefinite growth and allotted them only a limited span of survival. (Mature cells of a tissue are constantly replenished from a line of more primitive "stem" cells, themselves less subject to the changes of senescence, but subject once they have received the stimulus to differentiate.)

What if the programmed restrictions were removed, to allow cells to go on growing and dividing forever? We would then have the cells of a malignant tumor; there has been a genetic change abolishing restrictions on growth and multiplication, so that the cells have achieved autonomous growth. So long as the cells are provided with nutrients and a suitable milieu, in the body or in tissue culture, they need have no limits on their survival or multiplication.

The change from normal cell to malignant cell is genetic; there has been breakage, displacement, or deletion of part of a chromosome, so that certain of the programmed controls are abolished and behavior of the cell is altered. Specific chromosomal alterations have been identified in more and more human tumors, implying that some such change eventually will be found in all. Genetic information carried by chromosomes is coded in the double strands of deoxyribonucleic acid, or DNA. Strands may be broken by ionizing radiation, by certain chemicals, or in a few instances by virus infection. While some damaged strands of DNA may be repaired by the cell, damage not repaired is likely to be perpetuated in the cell's descendants and thus can constitute a mutation. It follows that a cancer begins as a mutation of a single cell, which grows and divides progressively from that point on. The visible structure of mutant cells also may be changed, so that malignant cells can be distinguished from normal cells under the microscope. Such microscopic identification is our primary method for diagnosis of cancer.

In the case of lung cancer specifically, the damage to chromosomes is caused by compounds from tobacco smoke, by ionizing radiation as from decaying radon daughters, possibly in a few cases by other factors. Some persons may be genetically susceptible to a certain type of damage, but if so, there is no way yet of identifying them beforehand. All the cell types of lung cancer bear a strong relationship to smoking history,[1] possibly with the exception of a fairly rare type, bronchiolar-alveolar cell carcinoma, for which the relation is less secure. Squamous-cell carcinoma and undifferentiated small-cell carcinoma are the common types among uranium miners, but these two also are closely associated with cigarette smoking.

GROWTH OF THE TUMOR

The newly mutant cancer cell continues to divide from time to time, but now the controls on its multiplication have been removed and nothing stops it. Time intervals between mitoses have been postulated to be roughly constant within the same tumor, implying that the tumor grows at a logarithmic rate corresponding to powers of 2. From this postulate has grown the conception of "doubling time," more accurately volume-doubling time, an index of growth rate in tumors large enough to be measured. Even malignant tumors show a wide range of growth rates, from very rapid to very slow; as one might expect, faster growth correlates with increasingly malignant behavior. (Readers interested in the concept of exponential growth rates and doubling times are invited to follow the argument in appendix A.)

Those malignant tumors technically classified as "carcinomas" are distinguished by the fact that they arise from epithelial cells. *Epithelium* signifies the thin discrete layer of specialized cells, forming a membrane which covers external surfaces of the body, or lines surfaces within it; examples are the epidermis or outer layer of the skin, the membranes lining the interior of the mouth, the intestinal tract, the bronchial tubes of the lung, and the like. The interior secreting surface of glands also is made up of epithelium. Cell types and patterns vary, so that different epithelial layers can give rise to different types of carcinoma.

A carcinoma originating within the thin layer of epithelial cells, and still contained within it, is called *carcinoma in situ*, growing "within the site" but without invasion yet. At this time it is not visible; it could be identified only by microscopic finding within a chance biopsy specimen. Continuing to grow, the tumor eventually breaks through the basement membrane which underlies the thin layer of epithelium, and from this time on it becomes invasive of the surrounding tissues. During a prolonged period of the tumor's life history, amounting in most cases to about three-quarters of its entire life, it cannot be seen, felt, or otherwise identified. It produces no symptoms and is in the preclinical, or occult, phase. Only in a few special circumstances could a tumor be identified while in this phase: possibly if it is located on the skin and is directly visible; or if it is located, say, on the uterine cervix, for by being at a surface it continually sheds a proportion of its malignant cells, where they may be picked up and identified in a periodic Pap smear. A cancer arising in any of the internal organs generally is not identifiable until it has grown to the size of at least a centimeter (four-tenths of an inch) in diameter. Common examples are a lump in the breast tissue, not usually palpable by an examiner until it is about one centimeter in diameter; a nodule in the lung, not visible on an X-ray until it at least approaches this size; and small polyps of the colon or large intestine, which can grow into cancer but are not readily identifiable below this size.

In the size range of up to a centimeter, cancers practically always are devoid of symptoms; also while within this range, almost all cancers would be curable by simple surgical excision. But few are found so early. Only upon growing considerably larger do most tumors begin to produce symptoms: some by bleeding; some by partial blockage of a bronchial tube, or of bile duct or intestine; some by causing pain from invasion of a neighboring structure; or by showing themselves in the presence of an obvious mass. Then it is late in a tumor's life history. The tumor already may be spreading by the time it causes symptoms, and the opportunity for curative treatment may be gone.

EARLY BEHAVIOR OF LUNG CANCER

During the asymptomatic, silent period, lung cancer occasionally may make its appearance in a chest X-ray film as a solitary rounded density in the periphery of the lung, the so-called coin lesion. Many persons have chest X-rays done even in the absence of symptoms—during a pre-employment physical examination, examination for life insurance, a hospital admission for some unrelated reason, or a periodic checkup by a physician. The coin lesion is only a shadow on the film, not a specific diagnosis; the same appearance may be produced by many processes other than cancer. When the shadow was not present on a previous X-ray study, and particularly if it appears in a smoker aged thirty-five or over, it becomes a much greater cause for concern.

Rarely, lung cancer may be detected when not visible on a chest X-ray, by cytologic examination of sputum. (Such tumors are said to be in the occult stage.) Cytologic examination of the sputum is similar to study of Pap smears from the uterine cervix. With sputum, there are limitations to the reliability of the method, namely: (1) a negative report, that is, a failure to find malignant cells in the smear, cannot be taken to mean that the patient has no cancer; (2) false-positive reports sometimes may be given, not very frequently; and (3) the method is labor-intensive with low overall rates of yield, hence not well-suited to screening large groups of smokers.

An occasional cancer, without having caused other symptoms, may plug off or obstruct the bronchus in which it originated; complete obstruction of a bronchus results in airless collapse or atelectasis of the portion of lung beyond that point. Depending on the bronchus involved, atelectasis may involve a whole lung, a lobe, or only a segment. Patients often note increased shortness of breath, beginning fairly abruptly, after atelectasis involves a lung or a lobe. Lesser degrees of atelectasis may cause no symptoms, or may aggravate a cough. Most lung cancers, unfortunately, are not discovered until they have begun to cause symptoms sufficient to make the patient consult a physician. Here is the especially adverse character of lung cancer: symptoms that do not necessarily mean incurability tend to be vague and nonspecific. Some coughing is a common early symptom, usually in the form of a gradual exacerbation of a long-standing smoker's cough, but even this may be absent before other symptoms appear. Small hemoptysis, a little bit of blood streaking in the sputum, occurs only occasionally in early disease; but such a symptom is more likely to frighten the patient into seeing a doctor. (Real hemoptysis, coughing up gross blood, unfortunately is common in late, incurable disease.) Only rarely, an intelligent patient may note a persistent localized wheeze, an almost musical resonance during inspiration, always felt within one side of the chest, and significant if it persists for more than a day or two. Very similar is the occasional patient who experiences recurring pneumonia in the same area of the lung, or whose pneumonia fails to clear completely under appropriate treatment. The localized wheeze, the recurring or nonclearing pneumonia all may result from a small tumor causing partial or incomplete obstruction of a bronchus; the area of lung beyond a partial obstruction is predisposed to recurring or persisting infection. So important is this consideration that physicians dealing with lung cancer say that any middle-aged or older patient, especially a smoker, who is treated for pneumonia but fails to show complete clearing of the lung infection, should be looked at very closely for the possibility of a small underlying lung cancer.

Beyond this point, hardly any symptoms occur that are not likely to be signs of incurability. Remember, however, that each patient is different from every other, that there can be exceptions to practically every rule in medicine, and that we can speak here only of probabilities, however strong they may be. Too often in the public mind, the symptom of cancer is pain. Almost everyone has had a friend or relative who died of cancer, and remembers the distress and unrelenting pain associated with late stages of disease. In the early stages, when it is likely to be curable, cancer in general and lung cancer in particular are painless. The onset of constant pain is an ominous symptom, signifying chest wall or mediastinal invasion, or spread to a distant site. Probably all thoracic surgeons have heard patients say, during discussion of surgery for a small but suspicious-appearing lesion, "But Doctor, it couldn't be cancer; I haven't had a bit of pain!" If the lesion is indeed cancer, and the patient has experienced no pain, that factor at least is in the patient's favor.

BEHAVIOR OF ADVANCING DISEASE

All the nonspecific symptoms may be intensified with advancing disease. A person may note increasing shortness of breath, more hemoptysis, sometimes more infection beyond an obstructed bronchus; this in turn may result in fever, chills, and malaise. Systemic, or bodywide, symptoms become more common with tumor progression, such as weakness and easy fatigue, weight loss, and loss of appetite. A very few patients develop symptoms of hormone secretion by the tumor itself; or if not hormones, of unknown substances affecting the body in other ways, as did Andrew Cunningham. Collectively termed the paraneoplastic syndromes, these take a number of bizarre forms, many of which are not well understood. Although generally adverse in their effect on the patient's prognosis, they are rare, and some at least of the syndromes are known to regress dramatically with treatment.

The progressing tumor may cause more severe symptoms by invasion of nearby structures, or by metastasis, spreading to distant areas of the body. The syndromes of local invasion include pain at the site if the chest wall is invaded; rarely, pain going down the arm if nerve trunks at the base of the neck are involved; also, sudden onset of hoarseness if a tiny nerve that controls a vocal cord is invaded within the chest. Invasion of another nerve may cause paralysis of the diaphragm, with increased difficulty in breathing. A striking change appears in the case of superior vena caval syndrome when the tumor, located in the right upper lobe adjacent to the mediastinum, invades and obstructs the superior vena cava, the great vein that drains blood from the upper part of the body. Then the patient's head, neck, shoulders, and arms become swollen, with engorged veins, while other veins forming communication to the lower body are prominent over the chest, just under the skin. Malignant pleurisy can result from tiny implants of tumor on the fine, smooth membrane which lines the inside of the chest cavities; these are likely to weep fluid into the pleural space so that the fluid collects rapidly and compresses the lung, causing progressive shortness of breath until the fluid is drawn off by tapping or by drainage through a tube.

The other mechanism by which the progressing tumor may cause more severe symptoms is by metastasis to other locations in the body. Local or regional metastasis to lymph nodes does not often change the severity of symptoms, but has a definitely adverse effect on prognosis. Distant metastases are likely to have been carried via the blood stream and, with only the barest few exceptions, indicate that the disease is incurable. The sites of distant spread may be anywhere in the body, but lung cancer has favorite target sites which include the bones, the brain, and within the abdomen, liver, and adrenal glands.

Metastasis to the brain may present itself in the form of personality change, increasing forgetfulness, persistent headaches, or confusion; later by gross alterations of behavior, loss of muscular coordination and control, sometimes convulsions, and finally coma. Early metastasis may be present without any symptoms, but when symptoms begin they are likely to progress rapidly. Spread to the bones may show itself as bone pain, often in the ribs or back. Later on, fractures may occur through sites of involvement, known as pathological fractures since the bone was already abnormal and weakened. Metastasis to the liver is common, often without much indication in the early stages. Later there may be gradual abdominal enlargement, vague abdominal distress, sometimes fluid accumulation within the abdomen, and jaundice, a deepening yellow color to the skin and eyes. All these potential sites of spread have to be examined during the initial diagnostic studies and staging. Generally speaking, definite tumor involvement at any distant site eliminates consideration of surgery for the primary tumor in the lung. There have been a few patients with a solitary metastasis to the brain, without findings of spread elsewhere, who have been cured after surgical removal of both the primary tumor from the lung and the metastasis from the brain. Such an outcome has occurred rarely, but just often enough that a radical, or aggressive, approach to treatment is justified in carefully selected cases. Solitary metastasis to the brain is a special instance. There is no other distant metastatic site of lung cancer where aggressive surgical treatment has been found beneficial to the patient.

In addition to specific symptoms listed, advancing disease results in progressive general deterioration; increasing weakness, weight loss, muscle wasting are common. Oncologists depend in their evaluation upon performance status as well as disease stage. A patient weakened, bedridden, and unable to care for him or her self has virtually no chance of response either to chemotherapy or other treatment.

Seven

WHY ME?

No answer has been attempted to the objection that if
the universe must, from the outset, admit the probability of suffering, then absolute goodness would
have left the universe uncreated. And I must warn the
reader that I shall not attempt to prove that to create
was better than not to create: I am aware of no human
scales in which such a question can be weighed.

—C. S. Lewis, *The Problem of Pain* (1940)

JOHN DELLACROCE. DECEMBER 1975.

John DellaCroce had called yesterday for an appointment, and now he
was sitting in the doctor's waiting room. He had not been there for the
past four or five years at least. At this visit he was frightened and depressed. He had been reluctant to come today, but it would have been
worse to stay home from work and worry. Finally he was called into an
examining room, seated on the table, and asked to take off his shirt.

Dr. Stanley Czarnecki looked through John's folder while listening to
his story. John was fifty years old and had worked as a meat cutter for one
of the chain markets in Lowell. Aside from having undergone a tonsillec-
tomy in childhood and an appendectomy during his teens, he had had no
significant illnesses. He mentioned a "nervous condition" in the past but
did not want to elaborate on it; actually this had consisted of an acute
panic reaction some fifteen years before, the result of a sudden combination of problems that now he hardly could remember. He had been seen
at a hospital emergency room, was allowed to talk out some of his problems, and was sent home with a few days' supply of a tranquilizing drug.
He had not kept the follow-up appointment but managed to stay on a
fairly even keel since then. He had smoked one and a half to two packs of

cigarettes a day for over thirty years. He was separated from his wife and children, lived alone in an apartment. He had not lost weight, and his appetite and breathing had not changed.

For years he had a smoker's cough in the morning, nothing much the rest of the day, but recently the cough had become worse and more persistent. About four to six weeks before, he had begun to feel some intermittent pain in the right side of his chest. For a while he tried to disregard it; but it did not go away, and now he was frightened. During all the years of smoking he had been sure that nothing could happen to him; after all, nothing ever had happened so far. Dr. Czarnecki could find no specific abnormalities during his examination, but arranged for a chest X-ray because of his symptoms. The X-ray films showed a definite five-centimeter (about two-inch) mass in the right upper lobe of the lung; also there was suggestive evidence of enlargement of the mediastinal nodes. Dr. Czarnecki was a general practitioner who did some minor surgery. He had John admitted to St. Joseph's Hospital in Lowell the next day and biopsied the lymph nodes in the right side of his neck using local anesthesia. The nodes were normal in size and appearance, showing no involvement by tumor. So far no clear diagnosis was available, in spite of the probability of lung cancer. Dr. Czarnecki advised consultation with a thoracic surgeon, suggested Dr. Bill Hunter in Boston, and got John an appointment in his office.

Readmitted at the John C. Warren Memorial Hospital, John underwent bronchoscopy and mediastinoscopy under general anesthesia. Biopsies taken from both sites were read by the pathologist as showing large-cell undifferentiated carcinoma of the lung. The next day, having received the definite report on the biopsies, Dr. Hunter stopped at John's room to discuss it with him. John was smoking another cigarette, and his ashtray was already half-full. He was upset and angry at the news, more so when Bill Hunter explained that because of the tumor cell type and the finding of spread to the mediastinal nodes, surgical treatment could not be considered appropriate. Bill always had made a point of plain discussion of the diagnosis and of the treatment plan with patients and their families; most of them seemed to appreciate plain talk even when the news was bad. This time, though, Bill felt he had made a mistake. Stress and worry had changed John's attitude to the point where he was ready to blame the messenger because of the message.

The radiotherapist who saw John began his consultation note, "Thank you for asking us to see this pleasant but deeply anxious man." He agreed that radiation therapy should be the definitive treatment and gave John an appointment to return the following week for the first session. John remained dissatisfied, unconvinced that he was getting the best advice or treatment. He had read magazine articles entitled, "Does *Your* Doctor Know How to Treat Cancer?" or similar disturbing queries, and was not sure whose advice he could trust in such an extremity. After he had pleaded for a time, Dr. Polzini agreed to call New York on his behalf, and arranged for an out-patient consultation at Memorial Sloan-Kettering Cancer Center. The Center had been mentioned prominently in one of his magazine articles. But the surgeons at Memorial examined him carefully, reviewed all the X-rays and reports forwarded with him, and finally said that they agreed entirely with the advice that he be treated by radiation therapy. Disappointed and apprehensive, John returned to Boston and began the course of treatment.

The following week Bill Hunter received a call from the office of Dr. Robert Wilson, professor and chairman of the Department of Medicine. The message was that there was a letter in Dr. Wilson's office that Bill would probably want to look at. Being from another department, Bill was puzzled until he saw the letter; then he remembered that this year Bob Wilson was serving in rotation as chairman of the hospital's Medical Board. The letter was handwritten on blue-lined paper.

January 16, 1976

To the Head Doctor, John C. Warren Hospital

Dear sir:

I am writing to you to ask that a reprimand be administered to Dr William Hunter. When I was a patient in your hospital recently Dr Hunter treated me with an entire lack of consideration, and his conduct was very unprofessional. The day after the biopsy he walked in and told me I had cancer and that nothing could be done for me. He practically told me I was as good as dead but not in so many words. I hope that he will be suitably disciplined because of this complaint.

Yours truly,
John B. DellaCroce

Bill read with dismay the reaction he had caused. If the news he had to tell a patient was bad, did that have to make him and the patient adversaries? The complaint was nothing—someone will have complaints or objections about any physician, and John's disappointment and distress showed plainly through the language. But John had sought to defend himself through denial of his own vulnerability, and by rejection of the adverse and potentially ominous news.

Later Bill Hunter heard that John had gathered up all his assets, after the treatments had been completed, and moved to Arizona. Almost two years after the treatment, John began to note increasing pain in the spine; tests showed recurrence of the tumor in the bones. He returned to Massachusetts to undergo additional radiation treatments to his back, then after consultation with an oncologist in Lowell, began chemotherapy for the tumor. The chemotherapy seemed to give little benefit but he continued with it so as not to miss any possibilities. He died in St. Joseph's Hospital in September 1978, approaching three years since he first had been found to have lung cancer; altogether an unusually long survivor for one who initially had inoperable disease.

WHAT DID I DO TO DESERVE THIS?

Many persons have smoked a pack or two of cigarettes per day for all of their adult lives, fifty years or more, and have died of some unrelated cause without ever having developed lung cancer. Others may be struck down by the disease after shorter periods of smoking, and at a younger age. Why me? The question expresses the bitterness of the natural human reaction. Why not, though? . . . Uh . . . Well . . . that sort of thing is supposed to happen only to the other guy . . . y'know, to someone . . . I mean, . . . someone who is less deserving, less of a special person . . . and all . . . .

Deep down, we all harbor such secret feelings, to which we would not willingly admit; but they may be jarred into involuntary expression by an unexpected catastrophe. Do they not enable us to hear of others' misfortunes, without feeling any unbearable pain ourselves? The feelings are part of our natural defenses. Certainly such affliction is unfair. If we say "unfair," we do not say who, or what, is to judge fairness or unfairness; or what sufficient Authority is going to concern Itself with the issue anyway. Most of the world's philosophers have wrestled with the problem. Do we have anything relevant to say about it? Probably not, but we are talking here specifically of our helpless anger and resentment at what seems to be the adverse working of fate, of our own subjection to a terrible disaster from which other persons have been allowed to escape.

Biologic scientists, virtually without exception, have joined the physical scientists in fiercely rejecting any model of the world, or the cosmos, which is determined by any but purely mechanistic principles. To admit otherwise in public would be to leave an indelible stain upon one's scientific reputation. If this view is correct, though, the cosmos is a blind machine, and we need not expect to find in it any concern for fairness or unfairness. In misfortune, the best that we can hope for may be some degree of concern from our fellow humans. C. P. Snow wrote some years ago:

> We should most of us agree, I think, that in the individual life of each of us there is much that, in the long run, one cannot do anything about. Death is a fact—one's own death, the deaths of those one loves. There is much that makes one suffer that is irremediable: one struggles against it all the way, but there is an irremediable residue left. These are facts: they will remain facts as long as man remains man. This is part of the individual condition: call it tragic, comic, absurd or, like some of the best and bravest of people, shrug it off. . . . Finally, one can try to understand the condition of lives not close to one's own, which one cannot know face to face. Each of these lives—that is, the lives of one's fellow human beings—again has limits of irremediability like one's own. Each of them has needs, some of which can be met; the totality of all these lives is the social condition.[1]

Finally some persons recognize a transcendent dimension to the cosmos which, in their belief, is accessible to the individual.[2] Is it easier for such people to find peace with themselves, at a time of extremity? All depends, we must suppose, on the person. Believer, stoic, or materialist, each of us may have to come to terms with illness or misfortune in our own way.

ANTHONY FEOLA. JUNE 1977.

Dr. Werner Heintzelmann felt tired out, as usual, at the end of the week. He maintained his general practice at the age of seventy-one partly out of a feeling of obligation to all his patients, but partly also because he could not imagine living without regular *Arbeit*. The Arbeit translated into a work load greater than most younger men could carry, but his patients of all ages loved him for his Teutonic accent and mannerisms, and he never was able to tell any of them to seek another doctor. He was talking now to Tony Feola, an old patient who had maintained reasonably good health over the years, but today was distraught and worried. Tony was sixty-one, a high school chemistry teacher in the Plymouth school system. He had been born in Brockton but had lived in Plymouth almost all his adult life. Six years previously, he had complained of periodic chest pains; Dr. Heintzelmann had him admitted to Jordan Hospital for observation and some tests, but nothing of consequence had been found. Tony had continued to smoke a pack a day in spite of the veiled warning. Recently he had suffered a fracture of a small bone in his right foot and had been treated by an orthopedist; the cast was off now, and he had been walking without difficulty. The minor injury had prompted him to see his physician for a routine checkup.

Tony said that he felt well, that his appetite was good, and that he had not lost weight; he mentioned some trouble with constipation. His wife was concerned that he had been coughing in the morning, somewhat more than usual, and Dr. Heintzelmann arranged for a chest X-ray. This proved to be the cause of Tony's worries. The X-ray demonstrated a rounded, somewhat poorly defined density approximately two centimeters in diameter, located in the left upper lobe of the lung. The nodule had not been visible on the last chest X-ray dated October 1975. What could it be, Tony demanded insistently. Was it cancer? Dr. Heintzelmann quietly responded that he didn't know, but that it could be; his advice was that Tony should have a consultation with a thoracic surgeon, and he suggested Dr. Bill Hunter in Boston.

Bill could see him on the following Monday; he requested as usual that Tony bring with him all old as well as recent chest X-rays. Tony was tense throughout the interview and examination, even hostile, although Bill could find no abnormal physical signs. The X-rays indeed were cause for concern that the nodule might represent a cancer. Bill explained the matter as best he could, and advised that Tony have several additional routine studies as an outpatient; then if these were satisfactory, that he be admitted to the hospital to have surgical removal of the nodule. Tony argued angrily against every point. Finally Bill suggested that he think about it some more, or get another opinion, but at this point Tony reluctantly agreed.

The operation went well. A frozen section confirmed the diagnosis of malignancy, and the left upper lobe of the lung was removed. No evidence could be seen of spread outside the lung. Having continued to smoke right up to the time of hospital admission, Tony was unable to cough in the postoperative period, and much extra effort by the nurses and respiratory therapists was required to get him to begin clearing his lungs. He remained feverish and short of breath for a number of days until finally he was able to begin coughing with some effect; then after the chest tubes had been removed, he slowly began to get back on his feet again. The pathologist's report on the surgical specimen identified the tumor type as moderately well differentiated squamous-cell carcinoma. None of five lymph nodes in the specimen were involved. Tony was discharged from the hospital after twelve days. No additional treatment was warranted because of the cell type and the lack of any evidence of spread; he remained vocal and dubious about this, implying that he had been written off without the "full" treatment since other possible methods were not being used.

At the first follow-up visit in Bill's office, Tony wanted to be told again at great length just exactly what had caused the cancer, and exactly what his prognosis was. "Smoking is the cause, Tony," said Bill. "Where have you been all these years? And why do you think we have been urging you to quit since before your operation?"

"Well, I'm familiar with research," Tony replied, "and I don't believe it has been proved that smoking is the cause. I've been inhaling ether and other fumes in the laboratory all the time I have worked as a chemist, and you can't tell me that's not the reason for my trouble. Who should know better than I what caused it?"

"If you see yourself as a researcher, and you have your answers all ready, there is no point in my arguing with you, Tony," said Bill. "You may be right about ether fumes, but if you are, there have been no studies that prove your point. We *do* know that smoking causes lung cancer, and no mistake. You have smoked for forty years, so which is the more likely?"

It was no use. Tony had resolved to blame his work exposure for the disease and would not hear of other explanations. Possibly this explanation was subconsciously more acceptable, not implying personal onus or responsibility, while he may have felt that to blame his disease on cigarette smoking would be to confess a weakness. At every office visit thereafter, Tony complained about the inconvenience of coming in, about the follow-up chest X-rays at intervals (he professed to be worried about the extra radiation hazard), and about various aches and pains which always were different. His antagonism and hostility grew; he kept a last follow-up visit with Dr. Hunter ten months after the surgery, but then no longer returned and did not acknowledge requests to make a new appointment.

In spite of all his worries, doubts, aches, and pains, Tony Feola remained without recurrence of the cancer. He couldn't help continuing to smoke but, more worried about it now, managed to reduce his consumption to half a pack a day. He retired from teaching and not long afterward, in June 1982, passed the milestone of five years since his operation—"D. F." or disease-free as Bill Hunter would have said.

Eight

DIAGNOSIS

I observe the Phisician, with the same diligence, as
hee the disease; I see hee feares, and I feare with
him: I overtake him, I overrun him in his feare, and I
go the faster, because he makes his pace slow; I feare
the more, because he disguises his fear, and I see it
with the more sharpnesse, because hee would not
have me see it. He knowes that his feare shall not
disorder the practise, and exercise of his Art, but he
knows that my fear may disorder the effect, and working of his practise.

—John Donne, *Meditation VI* (1624)

AN ATTITUDE OF SUSPICION

Part of the insidious nature of lung cancer is the probability that any
overt symptoms, the kind that are likely to make the patient see a physician, too often are already signs of incurability. But the doctor's dilemma
in this disease is to identify its existence as early as possible, realizing at
the same time that his diagnostic tools are expensive, inefficient when
applied to large-scale screening of persons possibly at risk, and even
injurious to the patient when over-used. Physicians are painfully aware
that early diagnosis and treatment are essential if we are to aim for cure,
but how are they to identify the presence of a disease that causes few or no
symptoms in its early stages?

Look for early disease among long-time smokers, most people would
answer. Who exactly is a long-time smoker? In spite of the approximately
twenty-year minimum lag period before most smokers are likely to develop overt disease, Andrew Cunningham and Elaine Schmidt developed

lung cancer in a much shorter time, and some other persons have smoked fifty years and more without ever developing it. For them, a screening test might have been repeated for many years, at considerable expense and with no return.

Only two tests are available that could be used to screen apparently healthy people for lung cancer in the period before symptoms: the standard chest X-ray and cytological study of the sputum for malignant cells. Each has its disadvantages and is less than perfect. X-ray study generally cannot identify a small tumor mass in the lung if it is less than one centimeter in diameter, or larger if it is obscured by normal shadows in the lungs such as those made by bronchi and pulmonary blood vessels. Each X-ray examination of the chest adds to the cumulative dose of radiation received by that person. Different cancers grow at widely varying rates, as discussed in Appendix A; so that no single answer is possible to the question of how often x-rays should be repeated in order to maintain effective surveillance. Because of increasingly straitened financial circumstances, health insurance companies rarely will pay for routine X-rays in the absence of symptoms. And finally, several investigations have failed to show that X-ray surveillance of large groups thought to be at risk (heavy smokers) has had any effect in reducing mortality from lung cancer. Cytologic study of the sputum is painstaking, occasionally misleading, especially in the presence of chronic inflammatory changes in the lung, not possible if the subject does not raise sputum, and ineffective even in the presence of cancer if for any of a number of reasons the tumor is not shedding malignant cells into the bronchial passageways. It follows that negative reports of sputum cytology, even several negative reports, cannot be taken to mean that the person does not have lung cancer.

A conference on lung cancer screening, sponsored by the National Cancer Institute in the fall of 1978, concluded that mass survey and screening programs had failed to benefit the study populations by any reduction of mortality. Subsequently, the American Cancer Society recommended, amid much publicity, that the routine chest X-ray examination be discontinued as part of the annual health checkup.[1] Many physicians have been dismayed by this pronouncement, Bill Hunter among them, for the simple reason that early, asymptomatic, potentially curable lung cancer generally is discovered in only one way—by identification on the chest X-ray. Results of mass surveys are not necessarily valid for the individual person who is found to have a nodule in the lung, causing no symptoms, but not present on the last X-ray a year or two previously.

It is possible that some reported mass surveys were conducted along less than ideal lines. Memorial Sloan-Kettering Cancer Center, with a favorable urban location, conducted between 1974 and 1982 a careful screening study of 10,000 male smokers and continues to follow the entire group; 354 in all have developed lung cancer. Tumors found by screening were more likely to be in an early stage, and resectable, than those discovered for other reasons such as symptoms or discovered after the screening period; also they were associated with a patient survival rate approximately twice as high.[2] Not surprisingly, the fast-growing tumors, especially undifferentiated small-cell carcinoma, were not reliably detected by the screening; and patients with them had poor survival. The combination of cytologic study of the sputum with annual chest X-rays was no more effective as a screening method than chest X-rays alone. But the possibility must still be considered that X-ray surveillance of people at high risk can indeed reduce their risk of dying of lung cancer, whatever the national societies have recommended. Surveillance can by no means abolish the risk.

INVESTIGATION OF SYMPTOMS

Failing early detection by screening, or by chance finding on an X-ray taken for some other reason, lung cancers can be discovered only when they begin to produce symptoms. As a general rule, if a cancer is responsible for symptoms that bring a patient to the physician, it will produce visible changes on the X-ray. There is no uniform or diagnostic appearance of lung cancer on the X-ray film; the picture is a collection of shadows of varying density which have no certain or automatic significance, but require interpretation. Lung cancer may take one of several common patterns in its appearance on the chest film:

1. A mass at the hilum, or "root" of the lung. This tends to be a relatively unfavorable presentation because: the tumor must have grown to a considerable size in order to be identifiable among all the normal hilar shadows; and at the hilum the tumor is located close to the lymph vessels and nodes in the mediastinum, and may already be disseminating through the lymph nodes by the time it is discovered.

2. Atelectasis, or airless collapse, which may involve a whole lung or one of its anatomic divisions, a lobe or even, rarely, a single segment, depending on the bronchus obstructed.
3. Recurring pneumonia in the same area of the lung, or pneumonia not resolving completely under appropriate treatment. Either manifestation results from partial or incomplete obstruction of a bronchus, which favors persistent or recurring infection in the area of the lung beyond the obstruction.
4. A solitary rounded nodule in the periphery of the lung, the so-called coin lesion. This is the form in which early, asymptomatic cancers are commonly discovered. A tumor presenting in this way usually is not yet causing symptoms, and tends to have a relatively favorable prognosis if properly treated by surgery.

Along with the plain chest X-ray film, other X-ray or radiographic techniques may help to identify and localize the tumor. Foremost among these is the computerized tomographic or CT scan. The CT scan is better able than the plain X-ray to identify enlarged, and hence possibly involved, lymph nodes in the mediastinum, as well as to identify direct invasion of the chest wall or mediastinum, and metastatic spread to the liver or adrenal glands. Finally, the CT is able to measure the radiographic density of tissue at any selected point; in the case of a coin lesion, a high density reading may signify deposits of calcium within the nodule, meaning that it probably was caused by certain chronic infections and is not a tumor.

Comparison of current films with old X-rays is of great importance, particularly in the case of the coin lesion or solitary nodule. Occasionally, old films forwarded from another institution may show the nodule present and unchanged, by measurement, for two years or more; in this case it is unlikely to be cancer and may safely be kept under observation. More frequently, a nodule cannot be seen on an old film, or may be present but was measurably smaller six months to a year before; either of these findings tends to favor the probability of cancer. If the last previous chest X-ray had been taken ten years previously and is clear, the comparison is not of much help.

X-ray and CT examination consist of images only, so that an exact diagnosis from malignant tissue is desirable if it can be obtained without too much difficulty to the patient. Cytologic study of the sputum may be diagnostic if positive but is inconclusive if reports are negative. Bronchoscopy is a technique of examining the interior of the larger bronchial tubes through a slim, lighted optical scope. Biopsies may be taken of any suspicious appearing tissue, and a biopsy report positive for cancer is diagnostic. Like all other tests, bronchoscopy has its limitations, primarily that it cannot examine all of the bronchial tree but only the larger and more proximal bronchi. Tumors located out of sight of the bronchoscope sometimes can be identified by brushing farther out in a small bronchus, or washing with saline; either method can yield special, selective cytological specimens. Finally, bronchoscopy often allows the surgeon to visualize the intrabronchial extent of a tumor, an aid in planning surgical resection.

Coin lesions in the periphery of the lung usually cannot be reached by the bronchoscope and, being small and far out, are unlikely to shed cells into the bronchial tree which would be identifiable in sputum specimens. Exact diagnosis still may be made by the technique of aspiration-biopsy through a long, fine needle passed through the skin into the nodule, using local anesthesia, with guidance under the fluoroscope. Again, the technique is not perfect, especially for smaller nodules. Institutions with a lot of experience find that if the nodule is two centimeters (eight-tenths of an inch) or less in diameter, even two successive needle biopsies may be reported negative in one-quarter of those cases in which the nodule is indeed a cancer. A report that the biopsy is unequivocally positive for malignancy is diagnostic, but a report that it does not reveal malignancy cannot always be relied on. So much is at stake for the patient that many thoracic surgeons omit any dependence upon needle biopsy if the patient's circumstances are otherwise suspicious for cancer; for example, if the patient has been a smoker; if the nodule has been seen to enlarge on serial X-ray films; if the nodule was not present, say, a year or eighteen months previously. In such cases, assuming that the patient can tolerate the surgery, it is better to settle the problem by removing the nodule surgically, than to leave it alone because it has not been proved to be cancer.

STAGING

By this time, a diagnosis of cancer has been proved, or there are grounds for a strong suspicion in case direct biopsy has not been possible. If the X-ray signs and the patient's symptoms are indicative of advanced disease, surgical treatment will not be a consideration because it will carry no possibility of cure. Then, further studies will aim to: (1) obtain a biopsy of some type to prove the diagnosis of cancer; and (2) prove that the tumor has spread outside the limits of complete removal, or if it has not spread, that the patient would not be able to tolerate the major surgery required. A specific diagnosis by biopsy remains necessary because serious decisions have to be made in the choice of second-line treatment, whether it is by radiation therapy or chemotherapy.

If there are not yet clear signs of inoperability, a careful search is made first for possible areas of distant spread. CT study of the brain, and of the liver and adrenal glands in the abdomen, is appropriate except possibly in the earliest lesions; also there is examination of the skeletal system by scanning after administration of a synthetic radioactive isotope, technetium 99. Positive, reliable abnormal findings from any of these studies unfortunately signify inoperability; there may be the sole possible exception of a localized primary tumor and a solitary metastasis to the brain if its location will permit removal without causing disability.

Next after distant spread is evaluation of possible spread to the lymph nodes within the chest, or invasion by the tumor into the chest wall or mediastinal structures, reducing the chance that it could be removed cleanly. Mediastinal lymph nodes often can be visualized upon CT study of the chest, and may be biopsied by the procedure called mediastinoscopy. Involved lymph nodes in the neck, or in the upper mediastinum near the neck, mean inoperability; involvement of a few lower mediastinal nodes without other signs of spread may not necessarily mean incurability, particularly if the cell type is squamous carcinoma. In selected instances of such involvement, aggressive treatment consisting of surgical removal of the tumor, cleaning out of the mediastinal nodes, and subsequent radiation therapy to the mediastinum may result in at least a proportion of cures. Generally, we have to recognize that mediastinal node involvement is an adverse finding.

If tumor spread or local invasion have not been found, the physician has to consider whether the patient can stand such major surgery. Extreme old age, frailty, or other disease processes are the most likely complicating factors; in particular, heart disease and lung disease. Some patients will be disabled by loss of the necessary amount of lung, but others are even worse off and could not survive removal of a lobe. Pulmonary function testing is necessary, an evaluation of the efficiency of breathing; also an evaluation of cardiac function and reserve since the operation will be a considerable stress. Those people having severe limitations may better be treated by some means other than surgery, even though their tumors might still be localized. Survival for the time being, is preferable to radical curative surgery which the patient does not survive.

Surgical treatment, then, offers the best available chance for cure of lung cancer, provided that the disease is truly localized, and that the patient can tolerate the operation. (We must make an exception to this statement in the case of undifferentiated small-cell carcinoma of the lung, in which surgery has limited if any usefulness.) An exact biopsy diagnosis is not always possible prior to the operation; sometimes it is in the patient's better interest to advise surgery on the grounds of educated suspicion. The aim of staging is to identify any distant or other spread that would make surgery inappropriate, in which case an alternative treatment must be chosen. All the studies used in staging are imperfect; virtually none can detect microscopic spread, but the medical profession can use only those tools that are available now. Staging studies also determine the planning of radiation therapy or chemotherapy. A short-hand notation for tumor stage has been devised called the TNM system (Tumor, Nodes, Metastases); it is useful primarily in research studies, for dividing patients into groups within which all members should have a roughly similar prognosis.

Nine

PRIMARY TREATMENT

Gentlemen, this is no Humbug!

—Dr. John Collins Warren (after the first
demonstration of ether anesthesia for
surgery, October 16, 1846).

Surgery is like the actions of a savage, trying to obtain by violence what a civilized man would obtain by
subtlety.

—Sir Berkeley Moynihan, FRCS
(later Lord Moynihan) (1865–1936)

SPECIAL PROBLEMS OF THE CHEST

Thoracic surgery, or surgery of the chest, is a specialty different from the other areas of surgery. What makes it different, and why should it have separated off from, say, general surgery? The reasons for its separation go back to the period after the discovery and development of anesthesia, deriving largely from the special character of the chest as the bellows mechanism for respiration or breathing. Think of an ordinary bellows, the kind used in a fireplace: when the handles are drawn apart and the volume within the chamber increased, air is drawn into the chamber; when the handles are brought together and volume of the chamber decreased, a jet of air is forced out through the nozzle. Suppose that a two- or three-inch hole is cut in the leather of the bellows and the handles are worked once more; the bellows mechanism has been destroyed, and air can no longer be moved out from the nozzle.

The chest with its enclosed lungs works in the same way. The rib cage functions as the two boards with handles, the diaphragm more or less as the pleated leather, the trachea or windpipe plus the mouth or nostrils as the nozzle of the bellows. In ordinary breathing, the rib cage expands and the diaphragm contracts downward; both these movements increase the volume of the chest cavity, and of the lungs at the same time, so that air is drawn into the lungs, the process called inspiration. Then the rib cage contracts, and the diaphragm is pushed back upward by abdominal muscles; as a result the volume of the chest, and the lungs, is reduced and air is forced back out, the process called expiration. The other organs within the chest, such as the heart, great vessels, esophagus, and so on, are much less sensitive to volume and pressure changes than are the lungs, and have no air inlets or outlets, so that they remain largely unaffected by the movements of breathing.

We must digress now to a consideration of general anesthesia as it existed in its early days, the middle and late nineteenth century. The first anesthetic agent used in surgery was di-ethyl ether, commonly known simply as "ether"; it soon was followed by chloroform which did not carry the risk of explosion as did ether. Both of these agents are volatile liquids but had to be inhaled as a vapor. To accomplish this they were dripped onto a gauze-covered mask held over the patient's nose and mouth, a method known as "open-drop" administration. As anesthesia was induced and the patient "went to sleep," respirations were depressed, becoming slower and more shallow. The special concern of the "anesthetist" had to be that not too much anesthetic be given; deeper levels of anesthesia depressed respirations further and breathing might stop altogether. So the anesthetist had to walk a fine line, keeping the patient sufficiently anesthetized so that the necessary operation could be performed, but not anesthetized so deeply that respirations or heart beat might cease. There being no electronic monitors in those days, depth of anesthesia was judged by eye and hand.

Crude though it may have been, the discovery of anesthesia revolutionized surgery. Together with antisepsis and then asepsis for control of infection, it opened possibilities far beyond surgery's previous grim domain of amputation of limbs to save life, of "cutting for stone" from the bladder, of care of wounds on the battlefield, and the like. Before the end of the nineteenth century, many kinds of abdominal surgery, reconstructive surgery on limbs, removal of the breast for cancer, and comparable procedures were well-known and standardized. To open the chest, however, meant instant death; planned and successful surgery within the chest lagged behind that within the abdomen by a margin of thirty to fifty years. It was not a question of skill or technique, but of a delay in understanding the special mechanics of the chest.

To understand why, let us return to the analogy of the bellows with a hole cut in the pleated leather. A similar effect would be produced by making an incision into the chest, specifically into the pleural cavity which contains the lung. Remember that the patient is anesthetized, already with respirations depressed, but now the bellows mechanism suddenly is destroyed and respiratory movements no longer move air into and out of the lungs. Deprived of oxygen intake and elimination of carbon dioxide, the patient can no longer survive, and promptly dies. (There can be a possible exception to this catastrophic outcome, if diffuse adhesions exist between the pleural surfaces of the chest wall and lung; these may hold the lung in its expanded position so that adequate respiratory exchange can continue, after a fashion. But then removal of a lobe, or a lung, would have required separating all these adhesions. Most normal persons do not have them in any case.) The story of gradual understanding and eventual elimination of these problems is fascinating. Those surgeons who were interested in the problems of the chest, and actively investigated them, formed themselves in time into a separate group and became known as thoracic surgeons.

Today the solution for this formerly lethal hazard seems disarmingly simple. Since the patient is unable to breathe spontaneously while deeply anesthetized, and with the chest opened, the work of breathing is done for him or her by reversal of the mechanisms. An endotracheal ("inside the trachea") tube is passed through the mouth and into the upper trachea after anesthesia has been induced; a small balloon on the outside of the tube gently closes the rest of the passageway, so that the patient's lungs and the anesthetic apparatus now form a closed system without leakage to the outside. The patient's lungs are rhythmically inflated and allowed to collapse, in a close approximation of normal respiration, using a gas mixture of the anesthetic agents plus oxygen. Now it does not matter if a large incision is made into the chest; the patient's breathing is continuously maintained, while blood pressure, heart rate, oxygen saturation of the blood, and other factors are monitored by electronic sensors.

THORACOTOMY

Thoracotomy, surgical opening of the chest cavity for the purpose of repairing or removing a diseased organ, is done in essentially the same way on either side, for virtually all operations except repairs of the heart and great vessels. The patient is anesthetized, the endotracheal tube placed, as are the various sensing devices for appropriate monitoring of the patient's condition. Respiration is provided through the endotracheal tube by a mechanical ventilator, or by rhythmic squeezing of a rubber bag by the anesthesiologist. The patient is turned onto the appropriate side, with the diseased lung uppermost, and secured in this position; the arm is moved up and forward so as to leave the chest exposed. The skin of the entire side of the chest is scrubbed for ten minutes or more with a germicidal detergent, and sterile drapes are applied that cover the patient except for the site of the planned incision. From now on, the entire draped area is rigorously guarded as a sterile field.

A long incision is made in the skin, beginning below the breast at the anterior end, extending around the side of the chest and curving upward along the back to a point between the shoulder-blade and the spine. The curve is necessary because the incision must pass around the shoulder-blade with its attached muscles, not over it. Two muscle layers outside the rib cage are divided, or sometimes one of the muscles can be retracted instead. All the little bleeding points must be controlled, most often by cautery, a high-frequency electric discharge which coagulates the tiny bit of tissue to which it is applied. The thin strip of intercostal muscle layer, between the selected two ribs, also is incised together with the pleural membrane just inside it. The chest cavity is now open. A rib spreader is inserted into the incision between the adjacent ribs and opened gradually, so as to allow satisfactory exposure of the surgical field. A careful examination is made of the entire lung on that side, also of the mediastinum for presence or absence of involved lymph nodes or areas of direct invasion by the tumor. A decision must be made at this time whether removal of the entire lung (pneumonectomy) will be necessary, whether the tumor can be removed cleanly within a single lobe (lobectomy), or even whether it is appropriate to proceed with the operation at all. Sometimes additional biopsies must be taken from lymph nodes in the hilum or mediastinum before the decision can be made. If it becomes clear that the tumor extends outside the limits of clean excision, cure will not be possible, and it is better to leave the patient with all the remaining lung than to remove it. In such a case, the operation is terminated at this point and the incision closed.

A specific diagnosis of cancer has not always been available prior to the operation. If it is not, a direct biopsy proving cancer generally is appropriate before the surgeon proceeds with removal of a lobe. Biopsy proof is mandatory before pneumonectomy; this operation is considerably more disabling in terms of loss of pulmonary function, and carries a higher mortality rate than does lobectomy. By consensus, pneumonectomy is permissible when: (1) biopsy proof of cancer is available; (2) removal of the whole lung is necessary to remove the tumor, but (3) there is no evidence of tumor involvement outside the limits of clean excision; and (4) testing has indicated that the patient should be able to tolerate loss of the lung and survive.

PNEUMONECTOMY

Assuming that all the above considerations have been satisfied, and that the thoracotomy has begun as outlined, the first maneuver in removal of the lung is to control the arterial supply. The main pulmonary artery is located in slightly different relationship on the right and left side to the other structures of the hilum, but on either side a careful dissection is begun at the primary hilum and the pulmonary artery is eventually freed and encircled. It is approximately the diameter of a person's thumb, with a relatively thin elastic wall which must be handled with care.

Every surgeon has gradually evolved his own operative technique, a composite of all the little details, methods, and maneuvers that he has found most useful in his own hands while operating. No two surgeons will do the same operation with precisely the same moves. Dr. Bill Hunter, for example, would do the operations as they are detailed here; he has retained a distinct dislike for some of the newer mechanical aids to surgery such as staplers, and concedes that his attitude often is regarded as old-fogeyism. Largely concerned with teaching and supervising residents, he feels an obligation to be sure that residents are securely grounded in the fundamental manual skills. "You guys will of course staple all you like when you are finished with training and out in practice," he often tells residents, "but while you are operating with me, you will have to do it my way."

With the main pulmonary artery isolated, enough of its length must be freed so that it can be secured at both ends. The basic technique is that it be at least doubly ligated at its proximal end, and once at the far end close to the lung. Ties potentially can roll off the end of a thin-walled elastic vessel such as this; the best precautions are to separately ligate several branches beyond the most proximal tie, or to oversew the cut end beyond the proximal ties. Either maneuver should make it impossible for ties to roll off. (Many surgeons prefer to staple across the artery with fine staples.) The artery then is divided, cut across, beyond the secure ligatures.

Draining from each lung into the left atrium are two large pulmonary veins, a superior and an inferior; these terms have nothing to do with quality, but signify upper and lower. The veins are short and broad. Each is dissected free, ligated doubly at the atrial end and once more at the lung end, and divided between the ligatures. Now all the large blood vessels leading to and draining the lung (collectively, the "vascular supply") have been closed off securely, by ties or staples, and cut across. The lung still remains attached by the main bronchus, and by folds of connective tissue in which numerous lymph nodes draining the lung remain buried. The node-bearing connective tissue is dissected free so that it will come away with the lung. The large main bronchus is isolated near its origin from the trachea, a gentle noncrushing clamp is applied across it, and it is cleanly divided beyond the clamp by a small blade on a long handle. The entire lung, now free, is removed from the chest and put aside; later, together with any other tissue removed, it must be forwarded to the pathologist for a careful, thorough examination including microscopic sections at all appropriate sites. The pathologist's report on the removed tissue becomes an essential part of the medical record, and a guide to further or continued treatment, especially in cancer cases.

Sutures to close the bronchial stump are placed under the clamp and tied after the clamp is off. (Again, many surgeons staple across the bronchus, and do not suture it.) The closure of the bronchial stump must be tested and proved to be air-tight. This is easily done; remember that under anesthesia, the patient's lungs are being inflated under positive (higher than atmospheric) pressure by the anesthesiologist as a substitute for the patient's nonexistent spontaneous breathing. So if a small puddle of sterile saline solution is deposited around the bronchial stump, bubbling will be seen with each inflation when an air leak is present, but none at all if the closure is secure. When secure, the bronchial stump must be covered by adjacent connective tissue sutured over it, which can form adhesions to the stump and give it some protection against breakdown or a subsequent leak. Now the entire pleural space is thoroughly irrigated with saline and inspected for any remaining tiny bleeding points; if present, these must be controlled. A count of all sponges and needles is made, and, if correct, preparations are made to close the chest. In contrast to the procedure after lobectomy, no tube is used to drain the chest cavity after pneumonectomy. The big empty space left by removal of the lung will remain, but no other lung tissue remains on that side to expand and fill the space. Instead, the space will gradually fill up with fluid which, being incompressible, has the effect thereafter of stabilizing the mediastinum and the opposite lung during the pressure changes of coughing or deep breathing.

Several intercostal nerves above and below the incision are blocked by injections of a local anesthetic agent, with the aim of minimizing the pain as the patient is waking up; the effect of these blocks is temporary, as any one knows who has been to a dentist. More prolonged blocking is possible by freezing the nerves, called cryolysis. Several heavy, doubled "catgut" sutures are passed around the adjacent ribs which had been separated, to hold them once more in contact and alignment with each other. In turn, the muscle layers of the chest wall, the connective tissues under the skin, and the skin are closed by suturing, the skin often with removable staples, and a sterile protective dressing is taped over the wound. The patient is moved onto a stretcher or bed, and transported to the recovery room. Depending on the patient's age, vigor, and state of pulmonary reserve, the endotracheal tube may be removed when he or she is sufficiently awake, or it may be kept in place for a day or two so that breathing can be assisted by a mechanical ventilator.

Following the operation, as after any major surgery, all the physiologic processes are watched closely: the function of the heart and the adequacy of circulation; respiratory air exchange and relative content of oxygen and carbon dioxide in the blood; blood replacement if necessary; volumes of fluid in and out, particularly the adequacy of urine output; return of consciousness and cooperation with instructions; relief of pain as needed; clearing of secretions from the lungs; and various blood chemistry determinations as appropriate. Patients are encouraged to get out of bed with assistance as soon as possible, usually the day after the operation, and to increase their activity in every way thereafter. After surgery on the lungs or heart, most persons can begin taking at least liquids by mouth on the day after surgery, and a solid or semi-solid diet within a couple of days after that. Depending on the patient's condition and motivation, many are ready for discharge from the hospital in a week or a little more after surgery, but older people often stay longer.

LOBECTOMY

There are a total of five lobes in the two lungs: an upper and a lower lobe on the left; upper, middle, and lower lobes on the right. The right lung generally is larger than the left, by a ratio of about 55 to 45. Not all lobes are the same size; the middle lobe on the right is the smallest in terms of its volume of lung tissue, the right upper somewhat larger, and the other three are of approximately equal size. The lobes are separated from each other, to varying degrees, by fissures or clefts between them, all surfaces being lined by a fine smooth membrane, the pleura. Each lobe has a hilum, a "root" comparable to that of the lung but smaller; the pulmonary artery branches, the veins, and the bronchus to the lobe all pass into it or leave it through the hilum. Also there are lymphatic channels leaving the lobe through the hilum, and lymph nodes as well; these are important markers in cancer surgery. Any of the lobes may be removed by itself, as can most of the pulmonary segments, anatomic subdivisions of the lobes.

After the chest has been opened by thoracotomy, any adhesions between the lung and the pleura of the chest wall are divided under direct vision, until the entire lung is free. The tumor is identified and its precise extent is determined, also the hilum and the mediastinum are examined for any signs of lymph node involvement. If the tumor is entirely confined to the lobe and can be removed cleanly by lobectomy, this operation is preferable to pneumonectomy. Dissection again is started at the hilum of the lobe, which in the case of the two upper lobes is near the primary hilum of the lung. The pulmonary artery, generally speaking, gives off individual branches to the pulmonary segments of which there may be from two to five in a lobe, and there can be considerable variation in the pattern of these branches, with which the surgeon must be familiar. The branches are isolated individually, freed from surrounding tissue, doubly ligated at the proximal end and once distally, and divided between these ligatures. The corresponding pulmonary vein must be freed in a similar manner, and depending on the portion of lung to be removed, the entire vein or its appropriate branches are ligated and divided. Now, after any remaining connective tissue has been freed and the lymph nodes dissected away, the lobar bronchus is clamped, divided, and the lobe, or specimen, is removed from the field. The stump of the bronchus is closed by suture (or stapling), with the same precautions noted in the discussion of pneumonectomy. Once more, the entire chest is irrigated with sterile saline solution, washed, so to speak, and inspected for any remaining bleeding points or sites of air leak from the lung. As always, the sponges and needles are counted, and all must be accounted for.

This time, the problems of management of the pleural space are quite different from those following pneumonectomy. Another lobe, or two, from that lung are still present; if properly managed, we may expect them to expand and fill that side of the chest, so that no empty space remains. But two things are necessary: constant gentle suction (negative pressure) must be applied to the pleural space on that side to bring about reexpansion, especially since there are bound to be small continuing air leaks from raw or injured areas on the surface of the lung; and the blood, serum, and pleural fluid which constantly seep into the pleural space must be continually drained away. (Collections of such fluid in the pleural space favor infection, called empyema, which can be a serious complication in the postoperative period.) During the days following operation, the patient will be most of the time in the supine position (lying on the back), with the head of the bed elevated at least some. Within the chest cavity, air will rise to the highest point and fluid will pool at the lowest. Usually, two tubes (thoracotomy tubes or chest tubes) are introduced through the skin and chest wall into the pleural space, the tip of one located at the apex of the pleural cavity, the tip of the other lying at the base of the cavity posteriorly. These are connected to a mechanism that applies constant, controlled gentle suction. There may be a modest, persistent air leak from the tubes for the first few days, and there may be considerable drainage of blood-stained serum and fluid, but these eventually subside. When the tubes have been entirely inactive for twenty-four hours, and the remaining lung is shown by X-ray to be well-expanded, the tubes are removed. All the factors of postoperative care are generally the same as after pneumonectomy, except that the patient necessarily is somewhat immobilized by the chest tubes as long as they must stay in place, and ambulation, or free walking, often must be somewhat delayed as a result. There tends to be less need for breathing assistance by a mechanical ventilator after the operation, if less than a whole lung has been removed, and strain on the heart is likely to be much less.

LESSER OR "LIMITED" RESECTIONS

Is removal of less than a lobe appropriate in the treatment of lung cancer? Seldom, but some patients initially have very limited pulmonary reserve, and already are short of breath at rest or with only the most minimal exertion. There are even certain patients with early localized lung cancer who could not survive lobectomy, let alone pneumonectomy. Since the early cancer, causing no symptoms, is likely to be curable because it is not yet spreading, its removal with just a small portion of lung may sometimes be curative. Surgeons speak of this as a compromise procedure, but limited removal can be done relatively quickly, and detracts less from the patient's remaining pulmonary reserve. To be suited for this kind of removal, the tumor must be small, located in the periphery of the lung or entirely contained within one of the lung segments. Segmental resection is done along anatomic lines, with individual ligation of the segmental pulmonary artery branch, the vein branch, and closure of the segmental bronchus. A tumor nodule close to the surface of the lung often can be removed by wedge excision, done without regard for anatomic lines by placing two clamps across the lung tissue in a "V" pattern, cutting out the wedge of tissue containing the tumor between the clamps, and oversewing or stapling the lung tissue held in the clamps. This can be accomplished very quickly, minimizing the time of the operation, but plainly it is a compromise form of cancer treatment at best, used in selected instances because of the patient's poor condition. After segmental or wedge excision, the pleural cavity is drained with two chest tubes as is done following lobectomy. An occasional problem with segmental resection is that air leakage from the lung surface, and therefore from the chest tubes, may be considerably prolonged.

SUMMARY

At the beginning of this chapter, I quoted Sir Berkeley Moynihan's comment about his own profession. It is true that major surgery for cancer is destructive, hazardous to life at least to some degree, often regarded as brutal in spite of all the refinements, and in the context of this discussion, only successful some of the time in its aim of eradicating lung cancer. For many patients, surgery cannot be used at all; some are unable to tolerate the physiologic stress, while in many others the disease already has spread outside the limits of surgical removal. Who would wish such treatment as this, and why is it not replaced by something more reasonable? Surgical resection remains the best treatment we have available today, for lung cancer in the clinically localized stage. What precisely does "best treatment" mean? It means the treatment with the best chance of cure; that is, of allowing the patient long survival without recurrence, five years or more after treatment. We may or may not be civilized, but we do not yet possess the subtlety to accomplish this equally well in any other way.

Pneumonectomy for lung cancer, in properly selected patients, carries a mortality rate of not less than 7 to 8 percent and generally higher, and lobectomy for cancer a rate of not less than 3 to 4 percent. Publications quoting a lower risk than these figures should remain suspect. A notable recent review averaged mortality rates between cooperating hospitals and quoted lower mortalities than any reported previously; but at one of the participating hospitals, the mortality rate for pneumonectomy actually had been 25 percent. An unresolved question remains: what deaths following surgery should be attributed to the surgery? The review in question included only those deaths that took place within thirty days of surgery, the so-called thirty-day mortality figure; but other reviews have noted that some patients may continue to die of delayed complications even after one month. A more realistic evaluation would include all patients who die before discharge from the hospital, known as the "hospital mortality" rate; this is found to be at least one-third higher than the thirty-day mortality rate.

Ten

SECONDARY TREATMENT

An archer stands up to the line, draws his bow, and looses an arrow at the target. The arrow first travels half the distance to the target, then half the remaining distance, then half the remainder, etc. It follows that the arrow can never quite reach the target.

Zeno of Elea (c. 490–410 B.C.); paraphrase of the third of four problems collectively known as Zeno's Paradoxes

Secondary treatment methods must be considered when surgical removal of lung cancer is not possible, or inappropriate; the two available are radiation therapy and chemotherapy. All this discussion must be qualified by the exclusion of undifferentiated small-cell carcinoma because of its fundamentally different behavior. Small-cell carcinoma will be considered separately in chapter 14; for it alone, chemotherapy and radiation therapy are the primary methods of treatment. This present discussion will deal with all the other histologic types, grouped together as "non-small-cell lung cancer" since the principles governing treatment apply more or less equally to all. The secondary methods imply treatment for palliation, or relief of symptoms, rather than for cure, except rarely when they may be used in conjunction with surgical excision.

RADIATION THERAPY

Ionizing radiation useful in cancer treatment may be in the form of megavoltage X-ray beams (energies of one million volts or more), gamma radiation from isotopes such as radium A and B or cobalt-60, or, more recently, electron beams from a high-energy accelerator. Radiation has damaging effects on all living tissues, most of all on those that are continuously regenerated from stem cells. Such tissues include the bone marrow, the white blood cells, cells of the reproductive system, and lining cells of the intestine; while tissues less sensitive to radiation damage include muscle, connective tissue, bone, plus the brain and nervous system. These are made up largely of mature cells with a low rate of replacement.

Exposure of the whole body to radiation is lethal at a dose much lower than can be tolerated by a limited area of the body; in the latter case, damage remains localized so that the majority of the body's sensitive tissues are able to survive. Dosage of radiation is expressed in terms of absorption of radiant energy by tissue, in units until recently called rads but now replaced by the unit named Gray (1 Gy = 100 rads). Many physicians who are not radiotherapists still think and speak in terms of rads. Malignant tumors, having a relatively high constant rate of replacement from their stem cells, tend to be susceptible to radiation damage; but unfortunately there are numerous cancers that respond poorly if at all to doses that the rest of the body can tolerate, and are known as radioresistant tumors. Even among radiosensitive tumors, not all the malignant cells are killed by the same radiation dose. Cell kill, rather, follows a skewed curve on a graph of increasing dosage, so that at first no cells are killed, then a few in slowly increasing numbers, then in rapidly increasing numbers at the middle range of dose (fig. 10.1). Now the more susceptible cells have been done away with; as radiation dose continues to increase, diminishing proportions of cells are being killed, and at last the hardiest remain which may tolerate a considerably higher dose and still survive. This characteristic makes eradication of a malignant tumor by radiation difficult, except in the case of the most radiosensitive tumors, or those small tumors located at a body surface where a much higher dose can be given than most of the host's tissues will receive. The curve of cell kill in treatment of a radiosensitive tumor would appear bent downward and toward the left, so that it could indeed intersect with the line of zero cell survival. In the case of a very radioresistant tumor, the curve would be bent upward and toward the right, so that it might never approach the line of zero cell survival (fig. 10.2).

A second problem with radiation therapy for cancer treatment is that its effects are limited to the treatment field, the relatively small portal, or area of the body that is being treated. The field must be kept as small as possible while still including the area of the tumor itself, in order to minimize radiation injury to the rest of the body. If the tumor has spread

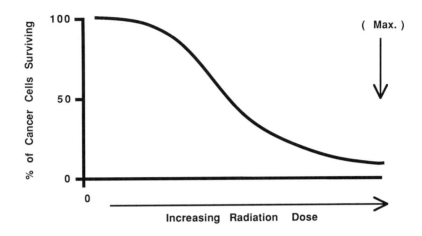

(Max.) :   Maximum Radiation Dose Tolerable By   Patient

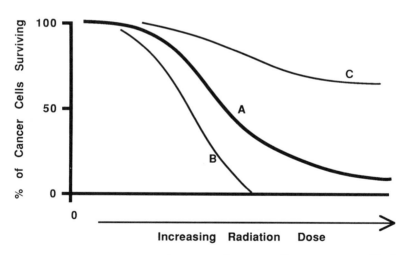

*Figure 10.2. "Shifting" of the curve of tumor cell response to radiation. A:
Standard curve as shown in Figure 10.1. B: Curve shifted to left
and downward, as in the case of a highly radiation-sensitive
tumor. C: Curve shifted to right and upward, as in the case of a
radiation-resistant tumor.*

to lymph nodes or metastatic sites outside the treatment field, these sites will be unaffected.

For example: a whole-body dose of 800 to 900 rads, or 8–9 Gray, given at once or over a few days will be lethal to practically all recipients unless newer salvage methods such as bone-marrow transplantation are used, and even these are not always successful. Conversely, treatment aiming for local control of the primary tumor in lung cancer must be given to a tissue dose of at least 5,000 rads (50 Gy) or higher. Patients can tolerate such a dose if it is given in fractions over a period of several weeks, and if the dose is delivered only to the area of the tumor while the rest of the body is well shielded. Dosage at this level is destructive to any normal lung tissue which is included in the portal; it is likely to cause troublesome difficulty and soreness with swallowing (radiation esophagitis) which generally is self-limited and passes off in time; frequently it will cause reddening, later tanning and dryness, of the skin; and most patients will complain that it has ruined their appetite for at least a number of weeks. On the other hand, radiation therapy is not painful nor particularly distressing in any way. Once begun, it amounts mostly to having the patient sit or lie in front of the machine for a short session, generally every weekday while weekends are allowed off. It carries little or no risk of immediate mortality as does major surgery, or of bone marrow depression or infections as does chemotherapy. There is some possibility of cure with radiation therapy, principally in the case of those cancers that have not spread but are not completely removable because of local invasion or fixation to other structures. The chance of cure in such situations admittedly is low, and impossible to predict, but still is present. A second situation in which radiotherapy may add to the chance of cure is after surgical removal of the primary tumor, when mediastinal lymph nodes have been found to be involved. In this instance, residual cancer cells are likely to remain in the mediastinum. The involved nodes are removed as completely as possible, but after the patient's recovery from surgery, the full dose of radiation therapy is given to the entire mediastinum. Such combined treatment is more effective in the case of squamous cell carcinoma than in the others, and least effective in the case of large-cell undifferentiated carcinoma. Disease may be controlled by this added treatment in at least a proportion of selected patients, who otherwise would not survive long.

Similarly, microscopic examination of the bronchial stump after pneumonectomy may show residual cancer cells at the level where the bronchus was divided, which could not have been identified by visual examination. (At pneumonectomy, the stump ordinarily has been cut as short as possible, so that no more can be removed.) Radiation therapy may be able to control the residual microscopic disease in this situation also, but if a microscopic residual of cancer cells is found in the bronchial stump after lobectomy, surgical excision higher up is preferable even though it may require removal of the entire lung.

Radiation therapy is useful in selected instances for palliation, or relief of distressing symptoms, when the tumor is inoperable. Radiation may be able to open up a bronchus that is obstructed by tumor, so that the remaining lung beyond is usable, and often it can control or eliminate hemoptysis, frequent coughing up of blood from an inoperable tumor. Radiation therapy usually can relieve bone pain from a metastatic site in bone, but by such a time the disease is becoming widespread, and pain soon may appear in other bones. Because of the problems of whole-body radiation dose, only one or two metastatic sites at most can be treated.

Does radiation therapy prolong life, in patients who have few or no severe symptoms and have no distant spread but who cannot undergo surgical removal because of mediastinal invasion, severe heart disease, or similar reasons? The best available answer is a qualified yes; there is modest prolongation of average survival when all patients are reviewed, but it is less than we could hope for. A few patients achieve markedly prolonged survival, but since they are few, their effect on overall survival is not great. The issue remains controversial whether all patients without distant spread who are not suited for surgery should receive radiation treatment.[1]

Postoperative radiation therapy can be effective for disease control in certain selected instances, when localized microscopic tumor residuals have had to be left after surgery, as in the bronchial stump, the mediastinal nodes, and so on. Why should radiation therapy and surgery not be combined in more cases, or as a routine? It was thought at one time that primary tumors too large to be removed cleanly could be reduced in size by initial radiation therapy, after which surgical removal might be successful. In several clinical trials, however, this approach has not prolonged patient survival,[2] and has resulted in more complications than did either surgery or radiotherapy alone. We must conclude that combination of the two methods is beneficial only when spread of the tumor is not a factor, but when a small and localized residual of tumor remains after surgery which could not have been entirely removed. Disease already spreading is a problem with which neither surgery nor radiation can deal, and patient survival cannot be prolonged by either method when distant spread has occurred.

CHEMOTHERAPY

Chemotherapy was visualized by its originator Dr. Paul Ehrlich, in 1910, as the "magic bullet" which would kill harmful cells or organisms while sparing the cells of the host. Developed first as treatment for infectious disease, in recent years it has had increasing effectiveness as treatment for certain types of cancer. Being a systemic, or bodywide, treatment, the magic bullet should be effective anywhere in the body, not subject to the limitations of local treatment modalities such as surgery and radiation therapy. But hardly any treatment in medicine comes so cheaply, unfortunately; and destruction of cancer cells can be accomplished, if at all, only at the cost of considerable toxicity or damage to normal tissues. Effective treatment for cancer often is a two-edged sword, involving danger to the patient as well as to his enemy.

The dramatic reduction in death rates from childhood cancers since 1950 is attributable at least in part to chemotherapy, but responses of the common adult cancers, including lung cancer, are less favorable. Only in the case of undifferentiated small-cell lung cancer is chemotherapy clearly beneficial for most patients, and in fact it is the key to treatment. For the remaining types, the question remains whether chemotherapy is of any benefit at all, but the issue must be examined closely. First, we should consider the theory and practice of cancer chemotherapy in general, then discuss its applicability to non-small-cell lung cancer.

Drugs useful against human cancer act by several different mechanisms, and are classified accordingly. The alkylating agents act by breaking and cross-linking the double strands of DNA, in which the cell's entire genetic information is stored; this group of compounds includes cyclophosphamide (trade-named Cytoxan), nitrogen mustard (Mustargen), phenylalanine mustard (Melphalan), and the nitrosoureas (lomustine, carmustine, semustine). Antimetabolites interfere with the synthesis of DNA, hence are active only while a cell is building the double complement of chromosomes in preparation for cell division; the most commonly used are methotrexate and 5–fluorouracil. Plant alkaloids are naturally occurring compounds found empirically to have anticancer effects. Vincristine, vinblastine, and vindesine are derived from the periwinkle plant, Vinca rosea; etoposide from the mandrake plant or May-apple, Podophyllum. Antitumor antibiotics are derived from molds, just as are penicillin and streptomycin, but these include doxorubicin (Adriamycin), bleomycin, mitomycin, and actinomycin-D (Dactinomycin). There are a few miscellaneous compounds, notably cis-diammine-dichloro-platinum (cisplatin or Platinol). (With drug names, we should note the convention that the *generic* name is written in lower case, but that the trade name, usually patented, is written with the first letter capitalized.)

While many of these drugs have their own particular toxicities for normal tissues, most are toxic to the bone marrow and the blood cells, the lining cells of the intestine, and other rapidly dividing normal cells. Limitation of dosage is necessary, and patients must have blood counts at weekly intervals after a treatment, with demonstration of recovery before the next doses are given. Patients may be prone to serious infections if the white blood cell count remains profoundly low for a period of time; during such a time they have little or no defense. Aside from this systemic toxicity, cisplatin can be toxic to the kidneys and to the middle ear, Adriamycin to the heart muscle after a certain total dosage is exceeded, bleomycin to the lungs, and vincristine to the peripheral nerves. These individual toxicities are less likely to be reversible after discontinuation of the drug than is bone marrow depression, and as a result special precautions must be taken during treatment.

Since the drugs act on cancer cells by several different mechanisms (not all of which are well understood), treatment with two or three drugs simultaneously tends to be more effective than with a single drug. Maximum tolerable doses of any single drug must be reduced by one-third to one-half when combinations are given. But the fundamental difficulty is that some malignant tumors are entirely resistant to chemotherapy in any form, while others are only minimally or occasionally responsive. Tumors that can be measured before and after treatment offer a method for gauging response; "complete response," or "complete remission," means that the tumor has disappeared entirely and no grossly visible or identifiable evidence of it remains. (Dramatic as such a response may be, unfortunately it is not remotely equivalent to cure.) "Partial response" is defined by consensus as a 50 percent or greater reduction in the product of two perpendicular diameters of a measurable tumor mass. In effect, this calculation reflects a 50 percent reduction in cross-sectional area, not volume, of the tumor being measured. Some oncologists record a reduction in size of less than 50 percent as "minimal response," and the finding

of no change in size after treatment as "stable disease." In careful research studies, however, such terms are unacceptable, and failure to
achieve the 50 percent reduction must be recorded as "no response."
Conversely, when effectiveness of chemotherapy is lost and the tumor
begins growing again, the term "relapse" signifies any reappearance of
tumor after complete remission, or an increase of 25 percent or more in
the product of two diameters after partial remission.

At this point we must consider the theoretical scheme of chemotherapy
effect on tumor burden borne by the host. Surgical excision amounts to a
one-shot removal of the tumor mass, which unfortunately fails to be
curative if there has been any spread of the tumor outside the area being
removed. We have examined the pattern of response to radiation therapy,
a skewed and reversed S-shaped curve of cell kill with increasing dosage,
often allowing survival of the hardiest cells beyond the dose limits which
the host can tolerate. Chemotherapy, no matter how successful, reduces
the burden of cancer cells by a pattern of first-order kinetics; this means
that a dose or cycle of treatment will kill a given percentage or proportion
of the cancer cells, never a given bulk or mass.[3] If the first treatment has
been effective, the total burden of tumor cells will have been reduced; but
at the next cycle, the proportionate rule continues to hold and fewer cells
will be killed, fewer still at the next, and so on. If the proportion of cells
killed by each cycle is very high, this theoretical scheme does not preclude
eventual reduction of tumor burden below the level of the last surviving
cell. Such a mechanism is responsible for those cures that are accomplished by chemotherapy. But if the proportion of cells killed by each
cycle is low, say 25 percent or so, treatment never will approach the stage
of the last surviving cancer cell. In the great majority of cancers, resistance to the drugs soon develops, at which time relapse occurs and
further chemotherapy is ineffective.

Suppose that a far-advanced incurable malignant tumor amounts
roughly to the equivalent of a single mass approximately 10 centimeters in
diameter, and weighs approximately a kilogram, 2.2 pounds. If the tumor cells average about 10 microns ($\frac{1}{100}$th of a millimeter) in diameter,
the tumor burden will amount to a total of about 10 to the 12th power
(10^{12}), or a million million cells. If each cycle of chemotherapy kills 90
percent of the cancer cells (assuming insufficient time between cycles for
regrowth to begin), three successive cycles will have killed 99.9 percent of
the cells, leaving a total of 1,000 million (10^9) cells surviving (see table
10.1). In this logarithmic scheme, such an effect is called a "three-log

TABLE 10-1.   Theoretical Scheme of Reduction of Tumor Burden by Perfectly Effective Chemotherapy

	Number of Tumor Cells	Tumor Diameter	Tumor Weight
(Before Treatment) →	10^{12}	10 cm.	1 kg.
	10^{11}		
	10^{10}		
("3-log reduction") →	10^9	1 cm.	1 gm.

(Complete remission, if it occurs, does so at this level, since internal tumors generally are not detectable at a diameter of less than one centimeter.)

	Number of Tumor Cells	Tumor Diameter	Tumor Weight
	10^8		
	10^7		
(2nd "3-log" reduction) →	10^6	1 mm.	1 mg.
	10^5		
	10^4		
(3rd "3-log" reduction) →	10^3	(1,000 cells)	1 mcg.
	10^2	(100 cells)	
	10^1	(10 cells)	
(4th "3-log" reduction) →	10^0	(1 cell)	
	10^{-1}	(tumor eradication in 90% of cases)	
	10^{-2}	(tumor eradication in 99% of cases)	

reduction"; the tumor has been reduced from a diameter of 10 cm. to 1 cm., volume reduced a thousandfold, and tumor weight also reduced a thousandfold from about a kilogram or 2.2 pounds to one gram or one-thirtieth of an ounce. A tumor in the lung cannot be identified by X-ray if its diameter is less than about a centimeter, so that reduction of a 10 centimeter tumor by more than "three logs," or three-log reduction of a tumor initially smaller than 10 centimeters, results in complete remission. Complete remission is not a cure. At this point, a total of three more three-log reductions will be necessary to reduce the tumor burden to the level of the last surviving cell, and more if the tumor is to be eradicated. Somewhere along the way, preexisting or mutant strains of cancer cells usually appear, resistant to the chemotherapy, and disease control is lost. Zeno's paradox could not be illustrated better than by the pattern of first-order kinetics.

Under all these difficulties, chemotherapy has the potential for achieving cure of at least some patients only in the most sensitive cancers: childhood leukemia; Hodgkin's disease and other lymphomas; some cancers arising from reproductive cells, such as testicular cancer; a rare pregnancy-associated cancer, choriocarcinoma; and a few cases of small-cell carcinoma of the lung. Used in conjunction with surgery, it may add curative effect in the case of some bone cancers and some cases of breast cancer. For the great majority of adult cancers, chemotherapy may induce a very rare complete response and a proportion of partial responses, most of which last from about two to five months before relapse (regrowth) occurs. Its proponents point out that patients who achieve partial remission survive longer than do those who show no response, hence it must be of benefit; but unfortunately this conclusion is not necessarily valid. All too often, if the responding and the nonresponding patients are grouped together, the curve of their combined survival will not differ from survival of untreated patients.[4] From a biologic standpoint, those who were classified as responders must have had the most favorable tumors, while those classified as nonresponders had the less favorable tumors and hence short survival. Unless a chemotherapy regimen (treatment program) can induce a high proportion of remissions, it may not prolong average survival at all in a group of treated patients; while if it induces a high proportion of complete remissions, it may begin to achieve a small proportion of cures. Against the too-free use of chemotherapy must be listed the problems of special toxicity, bone marrow depression, hair loss, and often the risk of serious infections. A final consideration is that chemotherapy is ineffective against metastatic lesions in the central nervous system, the brain and spinal cord; these areas represent a sanctuary for tumor cells against the chemotherapeutic drugs.

Non-small-cell carcinomas of the lung (that is to say, squamous cell carcinoma, large-cell undifferentiated carcinoma, and adenocarcinoma) are and have been notably resistant to chemotherapy. In many reports, partial response has been reported in as many as 12 to 20 percent of treated patients with inoperable disease, somewhat more with newer regimens, but with no proof that patients have survived any longer because of treatment. Only recently has a prospective, randomized study found evidence of longer survival with chemotherapy,[5] and for the time being this report remains unconfirmed by other data. Conducted by the National Cancer Institute of Canada, the study randomized patients with inoperable non-small-cell lung cancer to receive: (1) no chemotherapy but the best supportive care; (2) VP: vindesine and cisplatin; or (3) CAP: cyclophosphamide, Adriamycin, and cisplatin, according to maximum tolerable dosage schedules. Rates of response to the chemotherapy were low as usual (16 percent and 25 percent responses of any kind); while patient survival possibly may have been slightly prolonged by the CAP regimen ($P = 0.069$, not significant). Survival was prolonged by an average of less than four months by treatment with VP ($P = 0.022$) but at the cost of considerable toxicity: severe bone marrow depression in 40 percent of patients; severe vomiting in 12 percent; neuropathy (damage to peripheral nerves) in 15 percent. No cures were possible in the treated group. The dosage figures and the levels of toxicity confirm that these patients had been treated to their maximum tolerance; there could be no prospect of better response from changes in dosage or schedule.

Considering the possibility, not yet confirmed by other studies, of a bare few months' prolongation of survival, obtained at the cost of treatment every three weeks to the limit of patient tolerance and with much resulting distress, we must wonder whether the treatment really is worth while. This is an intensely difficult question, to which perhaps no two people would respond in quite the same way.

Eleven

SEVERAL UNSUCCESSFUL CASES

Nunc lento sonitu dicunt,
   Morieris.

Now, this Bell tolling softly for another,
   saies to mee, Thou must die.

. . . .

   All mankinde is of one Author, and is one volume;
   when one Man dies, one Chapter is not torne out of
   the booke; but translated into a better language; and
   every Chapter must be so translated. . . . As therefore
   the Bell that rings to a Sermon, calls not upon the
   Preacher onely, but upon the Congregation to come;
   so this Bell calls us all; but how much more mee,
   who am brought so neere the doore by this sicknesse.

—*John Donne, Meditation XVII* (1624)

ELIZABETH ANDERSON. JULY 1985.

Beth Anderson checked in at the receptionist's desk, then sat down in the office waiting room with her husband and son. She was fifty-nine years old, active and vigorous, a happy and outgoing person. She always had felt well and wondered now whether she had begun imagining some recent symptoms. When the secretary called her name she was taken to one of the examining rooms.

Dr. Gerald Hardy practiced internal medicine and had been her doctor for years. He had opened his office in Hyannis not long after she and her husband had been married and came to the mid Cape to live. He had tried for years to get her to quit smoking, to no avail. Seven years previously, in 1978, she had been treated for endometrial cancer (cancer of the internal lining of the uterus) by local radiation followed by hysterectomy, removal of the uterus. She had remained well and without recurrence thereafter. Recently she had noted the onset of a dry cough; in the last two weeks there had been vague pain in her left hip, and occasional vague discomfort in the right upper arm although she could recall no injury. Dr. Hardy noted that breath sounds were diminished in the upper part of her right lung. Nothing else was clearly abnormal. He had her go to Cape Cod Hospital for a chest X-ray, with the shocking finding of a very large irregular mass in the upper right lung field. Dr. Hardy also ordered a CT study of the chest and films of the bones of her left hip. The CT confirmed presence of the mass, showing also several enlarged mediastinal nodes, and a mass in the left adrenal gland below the diaphragm. The bone X-rays demonstrated a thinned-out spot in the left hip bone, suggestive of a metastasis. Dr. Hardy had to talk to Beth and her husband plainly and bluntly, saying that lung cancer was likely, almost certain; he advised consultation with a thoracic surgeon for biopsy and whatever additional tests might be appropriate.

At this, Beth recalled that she had gone with her husband to a convention in Chicago in December 1982; while there she had developed a bad cold with a racking cough, and finally went to one of the North Side hospitals where a chest X-ray was taken. The doctor had given her a prescription for cough medicine, but said also that there was a very small abnormal shadow in her lung. She should by all means consult her own physician about it when she returned home. Subsequently, the cold had passed off but she had been busy, preoccupied with her work and many other things, and she never had seen Dr. Hardy about it. The old film, obtained now from Chicago, showed a small, poorly defined oval density in the right lung, about one by one and a half centimeters in size, located precisely in the center of the area now occupied by the large tumor mass. The interval between X-rays had been thirty-one months.

Beth was referred to Dr. Bill Hunter for consultation. He was dismayed to see her like this, a delightful and likable person with such ominous signs of advanced disease. Biopsies at several sites would be necessary to determine whether one process or several were present, but all could be done at the same time. After discussion with her, he advised a brief admission to the hospital. The morning after her admission, bronchoscopy and mediastinoscopy were done, and biopsies from both sites showed undifferentiated large-cell carcinoma of the lung. Worse, a CT study of the brain revealed at least one, probably two, metastatic lesions, and a liver scan showed multiple liver metastases. All told, the tumor had spread by this time to brain, liver, bones, mediastinal nodes, and the adrenal gland. Neither surgery nor radiation treatment could cope with all these areas. Bill made arrangements for Beth to see an oncologist, who began her treatment with the combination of vinblastine and cisplatin.

Only three weeks later she abruptly began to develop increasing head-aches, lethargy, and confusion; plainly these were a result of the meta-stases in the brain, and she was given a medication which dramatically relieves such symptoms even though it does not affect the growth of the tumor. After urgent consultation with the radiotherapists, treatment of the brain was begun the same day, continuing for two weeks. She could not discontinue the new medication, but it allowed her to feel relatively well for the short time remaining. Beth died at home in early October, only a bare three months after she had first consulted Dr. Hardy.

What had gone wrong after the first X-ray study showed an abnormal-ity in December 1982? Beth could not recall exactly why she had not gone right away to see her doctor. She may have believed subconsciously that everything really was all right, and probably had a natural reluctance to worry about it. After the cold had subsided, she had felt entirely well. She was busy, and she could not believe, under the circumstances, that she might have a potentially fatal disease. Would the cancer have been cur-able then, if it had been removed soon after the first X-ray? It is impossi-ble to say with certainty, but at that time, the tumor was very small and entirely without symptoms. It had been identified early, and the best op-portunity for successful treatment would have been at that time.

JOSEPH MORELLI. JANUARY 1975.

Dr. Bill Hunter received a call from the Radiation Therapy Department at the John C. Warren Memorial, asking if he could come down to their office area in the basement to see a patient in consultation. Joseph Morelli was sixty-one years old, lived in Dorchester, had been a lifelong heavy smoker. In June 1972 he had been treated in the department for a cancer of the larynx; several lymph nodes in the left side of his neck had been involved at that time, but the nodes had disappeared after radiation treatment, and there had been no signs of recurrence. Unfortunately he had continued to smoke and had a chronic cough. About two weeks previously he had coughed up a small amount of blood. New chest X-rays at this visit had revealed a mass near the origin of the left upper lobe bronchus, which gave the appearance of a new primary cancer of the lung. It was not present on the last previous X-rays, dated more than a year before. Joseph denied having experienced any decrease in appetite, loss of weight, or change in his breathing.

Bill Hunter advised that he be admitted to the hospital for some additional studies and probable surgical removal of the tumor. At bronchoscopy and mediastinoscopy, no abnormalities could be seen; bronchial washings were interpreted as showing probable malignant cells. The other studies for distant spread were negative, or not abnormal, and a left upper lobectomy was done without any difficulties. The tumor appeared to be entirely confined to the lobe. The final pathologist's report identified it as poorly differentiated squamous cell carcinoma, with involvement of one lymph node adjacent to the tumor.

Joseph did well for the first three days following the operation, then began to develop vague abdominal distress and with it, increasing abdominal distention. Several enemas, intended to aid in cleaning out his colon, had no effect. By the fourth day, the physical signs plus X-rays of his abdomen were indicative of intestinal obstruction caused by volvulus (twisting) of the cecum, the first portion of the large intestine. This appeared to have no particular relation to the recent lobectomy, but rather had occurred at the time by random chance. It required immediate surgical correction to prevent gangrene and rupture of the colon; this was done on the same day by the consultants from general surgery. Thereafter, Joseph's recovery was slow but without further problems. It was another three weeks before he was able to leave the hospital. By late February his shortness of breath with activity had improved, he was eating fairly well, and he no longer felt any nausea or cramps.

By June he was feeling poorly again; his appetite was poor and he was losing weight and strength; he again had more coughing and shortness of breath. When he went to see Dr. Hunter in July, he was weak and thin. Dr. Hunter found his liver enlarged and knobby in contour, in all probability from extensive metastatic disease, and had him readmitted to the hospital. A liver scan confirmed the presence of recurrent tumor, although his lungs remained clear. A consulting oncologist advised that chemotherapy would offer him little or no chance of benefit. Joseph was allowed to return home with medications, and arrangements for a visiting nurse to come in three days a week. He died in early August, only seven months after first diagnosis.

Was the cancer in Joseph Morelli's lung a new tumor, or a recurrence of his cancer of the larynx which had been treated two years before? Only an estimate is possible, based on probabilities. First, smoking is the primary cause of both lung cancer and cancer of the larynx. The same carcinogenic (cancer-causing) stimulus is at work in both cases, and it is not unusual for a patient treated successfully for cancer of the larynx to develop lung cancer also. The two cancers had different rates of growth; the first one in the larynx had involved lymph nodes in the neck but had not recurred in two and a half years following treatment by radiation therapy. The tumor in the lung not only had the appearance and location of a new primary tumor, but it had spread massively to the liver in less than six months after surgical removal. In all probability, the tumors had originated at different sites, and their biologic characteristics and behavior were different although they had been caused by the same factor.

HAROLD CARSON. NOVEMBER 1980.

Harold had developed a bad cold about two months before, in September, and could not seem to get over the effects of it. He was forty-four, had always been in good health, and worked full time as manager of an auto parts store in Westfield, Massachusetts. His wife taught in the Westfield school system but they lived in Southwick. He had smoked two packs a day since about the age of seventeen. Ever since the cold came on he had had a persistent cough, productive of small amounts of yellow or gray sputum, and a couple of times there had been a few streaks of blood. He had lost about ten pounds of weight in two months. Also, he had begun to experience a troublesome and almost continuous headache which remained localized in the right side of his head. His wife insisted that they go to see their doctor about it, and reluctantly he agreed.

Dr. Maria Hassell noted his cough while talking, saw also that he was thinner than he had been and did not look well. The pupil of his right eye was possibly slightly dilated as compared to the left. There were a few rales, fine crackling sounds during breathing, in the lateral and anterior portions of his left lung. There were no painful or tender spots in his bones, and no sign that his liver was enlarged. His fingers showed definite clubbing, although he had not complained of painful or swollen joints. Concerned about his cough, the blood streaking in the sputum, and his smoking history, Dr. Hassell arranged for him to have a chest X-ray, and after it was found to be abnormal, a CT study of the chest. Both studies demonstrated an irregular mass in the left upper lobe about five centimeters (two inches) in diameter, with evidence of extension toward the hilum of the lung. Dr. Hassell had been the Carson's doctor for years and knew them both well. It was doubly hard to talk to them bluntly and break such bad news, but she said that the problem appeared to be lung cancer, and she wanted to refer Harold to Boston for further studies and treatment. Plainly he needed to be in a hospital very soon; she made an appointment for him to be admitted to the John C. Warren Memorial in two days.

In the hospital, the admission laboratory tests were normal. Bronchoscopy and mediastinoscopy on the morning after admission found no abnormalities, except that bronchial washings were called suspicious for the presence of malignant cells. A CT study of the brain demonstrated two, possibly three, lesions on the right side which had the appearance of metastases. No exact diagnosis was available yet; but an aspiration-needle biopsy of the lung mass under fluoroscopy was called positive for malignant cells, undifferentiated large-cell carcinoma in type. There could be no consideration of surgical treatment. The brain metastases and the progressive headaches were danger signs. Harold was given a tiny pill four times a day, called Decadron, which completely relieved his headaches although it was known to do nothing against the cancer. Consultation was arranged with the radiotherapists who agreed that treatment should be given to both sites, the brain and the primary tumor in the lung. Harold could not stay in the hospital for several weeks of treatment and Southwick was a long way from Boston, too far to travel on a daily basis. Arrangements were made for him to have his treatments at the Baystate Medical Center in Springfield, closer to home, and he was discharged from the hospital.

The radiotherapist planned a treatment course of relative severity, with the hope of relieving his symptoms for as long as possible. Treatment lasted for seven weeks in all, finishing in mid-January of 1981. Total radiation dose to the brain amounted to 4,000 rads or "centi-Gray," and to the tumor in the chest to 5,700 cGy. By the time Harold had recovered from the treatments, he was gradually able to discontinue the Decadron pills, and remained free of headaches for a number of months. He found it impossible to return to work on a full time basis; he was too fatigued after just a few hours on the job and finally gave it up.

In late July he began to notice pain in his lower back and going down both legs; it grew progressively worse instead of better, and in early

August he returned to see the radiotherapist before his scheduled follow-up appointment. Recurrent disease was found in the lower spine and in the hip bones, for which he was given additional radiation treatment with the hope of relieving his pain. From that time on he lost weight and strength more rapidly. Dr. Hassell had him admitted to Noble Hospital as his condition approached a terminal state, and he died in September of 1981.

For a patient who had had brain metastases at the time of diagnosis, Harold had survived for an unusually long time, about ten months. There might have been two possible explanations: first, that the tumor had been an unusually slowly-growing one. This is unlikely since he had experienced symptoms only for a bare two months before diagnosis, at which time metastases to the brain were already present; such a sequence suggests very rapid tumor growth. More likely, he had had an unusually good response to radiation therapy, better than most for non-small-cell carcinoma. The radiation dose he was given to the brain was quite high, more than some patients can tolerate without injury; but in this case the radiotherapist probably did right to have treated him with relative severity.

RICHARD WOLFE. MARCH 1978.

At work this morning, Richard Wolfe had accidentally fallen backward and hit the right side of his chest against a table; the pain was intense and he was sure he must have broken a couple of ribs. He asked his supervisor for permission to go to sick call at the station dispensary and, once there, was sent to the X-ray department for a chest film and spot films of rib detail in the area of soreness. The verdict after review of the X-rays was that no rib fractures could be seen, but unexpectedly the chest film had revealed a mass in his left lung. He was given an appointment to return later in the week to see a consulting physician who was coming on that day.

Richard was sixty-three, a machinist working in the North Slope oil field in Alaska, nearing retirement age but hoping to keep working as long as he could because of the pay scale for hardship duty at remote installations. He had been a heavy smoker since his early teens but otherwise had been in fairly good health. When he went back to the clinic the consultant, Dr. Julian, queried him in detail about his past medical history. Richard denied having experienced any new or unusual symptoms, but admitted to having had a cough recently. Except for the soreness in his ribs, resulting from the accident, Dr. Julian could find no particularly abnormal physical signs; a small one-centimeter lymph node could be felt at the base of his right neck, of uncertain significance. He advised Richard to obtain leave and return to the "Outside" to seek consultation and treatment. It was a couple of weeks before Richard could arrange for his replacement and get air passage to Seattle. He brought with him the X-rays from Alaska.

Richard's home was in Keene, New Hampshire, where his wife still worked for the county clerk's office. They went together to see their doctor. The pain in his ribs was diminishing now, almost gone, but the cough had persisted. A new chest X-ray, after an interval of nearly three weeks, did not differ in appearance from the first one. The doctor said that the mass probably represented lung cancer, and suggested that Richard go to Boston for diagnosis and treatment. Through Dr. Bill Hunter's office, he got an appointment for Richard's admission to the hospital on the following Sunday.

In the hospital, Bill Hunter reviewed the first and most recent X-ray films. The mass was fairly large, about five centimeters in diameter, located near the apex of the left upper lobe. It would be out of reach of visualization by bronchoscopy. There was no visible sign of any extension, but Bill scheduled him for mediastinoscopy on the morning after admission. When no abnormal mediastinal nodes could be found, he removed the small node at the base of the right neck as a biopsy; this showed reactive changes in the lymph node but no sign of tumor involvement. Scans of the liver, bones, and brain revealed no abnormalities, and tests of his breathing capacity were adequate. Bill discussed the problem at length with Richard and his wife, advising that surgical resection should be done if feasible. They agreed and asked him to proceed.

Richard tolerated the operation fairly well, although he had continued to smoke right up until that day. The left upper lobe was removed without any difficulties. During the few days after the operation he was unable to cough or to breathe deeply; secretions accumulated in his lungs leading to persistent fever and diffuse infection, and not until after a few days of vigorous tracheal suctioning was he able to cough effectively once more. Thereafter his condition gradually improved, he began ambulation, and was discharged from the hospital on the thirteenth day after surgery. Two weeks after discharge he was doing well, with only minimal soreness remaining. His breathing was good and his appetite had improved. He wanted permission to return to work in the Far North, but on Bill's advice agreed to wait another three weeks.

In late January 1979 he returned from Alaska to see Dr. Hunter. He was visibly pale and rather weak. Since about November he had noticed gradual swelling of his arms, shoulders, and neck, together with pain that had gradually increased. His voice had become hoarse at about the same time. His appetite had been poor, and he had lost nine or ten pounds since October. New chest X-rays revealed a large mass of recurrent tumor in the upper mediastinum; plainly the mass was the cause of vocal cord paralysis as well as superior vena caval syndrome. Radiation therapy to the recurrent tumor mass was begun, which in time relieved his pain for a period of several months. Back home, he never was capable of much activity. His weakness and weight loss gradually increased. In September he was approaching a terminal state, and once more was suffering from constant and increasing pain. His doctor readmitted him to the hospital in Keene, where he died at the end of September.

Adverse factors of lifestyle, tensions on the job, and the like are some of the obstacles to quitting smoking, and thus to reducing lung cancer risk. Was Richard Wolfe at a disadvantage because of such pressures? He had smoked since his teens, but in those days smoking had not been regarded as any problem. We have no information about whether he had tried to quit during adult life, or even whether he had wanted to. Isolation, boredom, loneliness, separation from family all are powerful factors tending to perpetuate the smoking habit; Richard was subject to them all. It's doubtful if once addicted, anyone could have quit under such conditions, no matter how strong his resolve. Military veterans of World War II, Korea, and Vietnam contracted the cigarette addiction in massive numbers. In civilian life, before the period of approximately 1958 to 1960, persons found to have tuberculosis had to enter a sanatorium for treatment, a stay that might last a year or several years. It was almost impossible for them to escape addiction to cigarettes, and sanatorium physicians recognized the frequency of lung cancer as a secondary disease.

THOMAS ANDERSON. APRIL 1974.

Thomas Anderson, no relation to Beth, was a slight acquaintance of Bill Hunter's; they both were members at the old Emmanuel Church on Newbury Street, in the Back Bay. Tom had been a vestryman before Bill and his family had joined, later a trustee as well. They seldom met at any other time. Bill was aware that Tom was a graduate of West Point, had left the army some years before, and now was a vice president of the John Hancock Mutual Life Insurance Company. On leaving the army he had transferred his commission into the Massachusetts National Guard. He often came to church in uniform, two stars on each shoulder, before spending the rest of Sunday with the headquarters unit on Commonwealth Avenue. Bill learned later that he commanded the Guard's Twenty-Sixth Infantry Division; the division had gradually shrunk in size over the years since World War II and now was at hardly more than the strength of a brigade.

More noticeable than his uniform on Sunday mornings was Tom's habit along with two or three of his friends of lighting up their cigarettes the moment they emerged from church. Bill Hunter was aware of Tom's habit partly because he still was a hopeless addict himself; most of the time, however, he could do without lighting up at least until he was on the way home. He had no idea of Tom's total daily consumption. One day Bill was shocked to learn that Tom Anderson had been found to have lung cancer and could not undergo surgery; he was being treated by radiation therapy at a prestigious private clinic in Burlington. In five months Tom was dead; he had been only fifty-eight.

Tom had smoked moderately since high school, none at the Academy, but had acquired his real addiction while a company-grade officer during World War II. Periods of tension, fear, and long stretches of boredom had had their effect, as they did on everyone else. In the forward areas, cigarettes had been distributed freely, along with rations; while in the rear areas or at the stateside camps they were a nickel a pack at the officers' club. Even after the war was over, there had been no Surgeon General's Report to warn of the hazards of smoking—that would not appear for almost twenty years—or of the risk of becoming addicted.

VIRGINIA HADLEY. AUGUST 1972.

Bill Hunter was seeing an elderly lady patient, Mrs. Virginia Hadley from Beverly, Massachusetts, at her first office visit. Mrs. Hadley was seventy-four, widowed, and still lived in her house by herself. She had been in fairly good health, except for heart trouble for which she had been taking digoxin and a fluid pill daily for about six years. For four to five months she had been troubled by increasing cough and shortness of breath. Also she tired more easily than usual and had lost several pounds.

Two weeks previously she had coughed up a little blood and, as a result, went to her doctor who had chest X-rays taken. He told her that he was concerned about the findings and wanted her to go in to Boston for a consultation. She had never smoked.

This last statement, spoken with quiet conviction but no special emphasis, concerned Bill Hunter as he listened to her story. He could not possibly doubt what she said. The films she had brought in with her gave every indication that her problem was lung cancer; the area of the right hilum was enlarged, and there was atelectasis or airless collapse of the right upper lobe indicating obstruction of the right upper lobe bronchus. Physical examination suggested no other sites of invovement. CT study had not yet been developed. Bill arranged for her to be admitted to the hospital for biopsies and some tests, to which she readily agreed.

Bronchoscopy and mediastinoscopy were done first. Through the bronchoscope, Bill could see a tumor mass obstructing the right upper lobe bronchus, as expected, and obtained biopsies. At mediastinoscopy he encountered some enlarged hard nodes high in the mediastinum and took biopsies of these also. Tissue obtained from both sites was read within a day as showing moderately well differentiated squamous cell carcinoma. Brain, liver, and bone scans failed to show extension of the tumor to these areas.

Mrs. Hadley's problem was difficult and unexpected. Was there any possible way she could be treated with hope of cure? Already she was elderly, with a history of heart disease for which she had taken medication for several years, but now it was found that she not only had lung cancer but extensive involvement of the mediastinal nodes. All recorded experience confirmed that there could be little or no possibility of cure; in view of her age and heart disease it was unlikely that she could survive removal of the whole lung in any case. Bill talked over the entire problem with her, in plain terms, and advised that she be treated by radiation therapy. He suggested also that if she wished, she could get a second opinion, but she immediately dismissed the idea and said that she would be happy to do whatever he advised. Her treatment schedule was planned after the usual consultation. Arrangements were made for American Cancer Society volunteers to drive her in to Boston every day for the treatments, and she was allowed to go home. She returned to the care of her own doctor. Bill Hunter learned only much later that she had died at home, about eight months after the first office visit to see him.

How could it be that Mrs. Hadley, a lifelong nonsmoker, had died of lung cancer? Different reviews have found that 92 to 96 percent of people who develop squamous cell carcinoma of the lung are or have been heavy smokers. Was it possible that her house was infiltrated by radon seepage? Possibly, but her illness occurred long before the radon risk in homes was known or had become a source of concern. Could her late husband have been a heavy smoker, and could she have been exposed secondhand? Again, possibly; the hazard of second-hand smoke exposure had not been recognized at the time of her illness, and she had not been questioned about it. Her medical history recorded that her husband had died of a heart attack, but his smoking habits were not stated.

Twelve

SEVERAL SUCCESSFUL CASES

And do not say, regarding any thing, "I am going to do
that tomorrow"; say only, "Insh'allah; if God will."

—The Koran, Sura 18: 23–24

Rejoice, we are victorious.

—Pheidippides (last words, after having run
from Marathon to Athens, 490 B.C.)

ALFREDO BARDUCCI. FEBRUARY 1964.

Last August Alfredo Barducci had gone to a neighborhood street fair in
Charlestown, not far from where he lived. At the time, the Health Department made a practice of sending its mobile X-ray unit to as many
festivals and gatherings as possible, to offer free mini chest films as part of
its inner city survey program for tuberculosis. Passing by the van, Alfredo and his wife went in, gave their names, and had the films taken in
just a few minutes. A week later cards arrived in the mail, saying that her
film was all right but that Alfredo's was abnormal; he was requested to
see his own physician for follow-up.

Both the survey mini film and a new full sized chest X-ray showed a
poorly defined density in the left upper lobe. The appearance of the
density was nonspecific; it could have represented any one of a number of
disease processes. Alfredo was fifty-five, had emigrated to the United
States as a young man in the late 1920s. He worked at a steel processing
plant and had been subjected to smoke and fumes over the years. He had
smoked for many years but had quit three years previously. He was
known to be a mild diabetic but required no medication. There had been
an eye injury during childhood which left his right eye of little use. He

had no symptoms currently. His doctor applied a tuberculin skin test which was strongly positive, meaning only that he had contracted infection by TB organisms at some time in his life. Two sputum specimens were read as negative for acid-fast bacilli and for malignant cells. He was begun on treatment with a single drug, Isoniazid, largely on grounds of the positive skin test without TB organisms in his sputum.

Follow-up chest X-rays had been scheduled at six months, in early February; to his doctor's concern, they showed the shadow in his lung to be distinctly larger. More worrisome, though, was a new lumpy shadow at the left hilum which had not been apparent on the previous films. The change in appearance, the progression, now suggested lung cancer with involvement of a large hilar node. His physician told Alfredo that he would have to get him an appointment for consultation with a thoracic surgeon.

Dr. Bill Hunter was new at the John C. Warren Memorial at this time, the most junior member of the thoracic surgery staff, and the consultation request landed with him. After seeing Alfredo for the first office visit, he advised admission to the hospital for some biopsies and tests, and probable surgical removal. (This was long before the time of harsh restrictions on days in the hospital for surgical patients.) Admission laboratory studies were unremarkable except for a moderately high blood sugar, consistent with his known diabetes, and the finding of atypical cells in his sputum which could not be clearly identified as malignant. Bronchoscopy and biopsy of the lymph nodes at the base of the neck on the left were unrevealing (mediastinoscopy also was not being done yet), so that a specific diagnosis was not available. This was one of the instances in which a strong suspicion of cancer, an educated guess, had to be the grounds for advising surgical removal. Bill discussed the problem at length with Alfredo and his wife; they agreed that he should proceed with the operation as soon as it could be scheduled.

The upper lobe was removed without difficulty. There was a very large hard lymph node, about the diameter of a quarter, wedged into the mediastinum in the cleft known to surgeons as the aorto-pulmonary recess. Biopsy of the node and frozen section established that it indeed was involved by cancer. No other nodes could be found. Bill found that the node could be separated from the large blood vessels on either side but that to remove it he would have to sacrifice the tiny nerve that controls the left vocal cord. Although this would leave the patient permanently hoarse, he did it without hesitation. Alfredo tolerated the operation well except for difficulty in clearing his lung secretions for the first few days, and some resultant fever, but otherwise made a satisfactory recovery. His voice was hoarse as expected. The pathologist's report called the tumor poorly differentiated, probably adenocarcinoma in type; the large node was replaced by tumor but none of the other hilar nodes in the specimen were involved. Alfredo was discharged home on the twelfth day after surgery. At this time it was not yet accepted practice to treat the mediastinum with radiation therapy unless gross residual tumor was known to have been left behind; as a result he received no further treatment. Bill saw him in the office for several follow-up visits, after which Alfredo returned to the care of his family doctor.

In the years that followed, Bill Hunter received occasional notes from Alfredo's doctor about him, and saw him once because of complaints of moderate shortness of breath with exertion. His voice remained hoarse but he did not seem to mind. He had retired from work and remained active and cheerful. The last time Bill saw him was twenty-four years after the operation; there was an overwhelming feeling of déjà vu on seeing his face and hearing his voice, considering all that had gone before. Age was adding to Alfredo's disability by this time and he was becoming thinner, more short of breath, but still he had achieved phenomenal survival after surgery for lung cancer.

He had presented initially with involvement of a mediastinal node, ordinarily a sign of virtual incurability, but in fact he had achieved a normal life expectancy after treatment. Not until many years after this operation did Bill Hunter see a paper in one of the thoracic surgical journals, finding that lymph node involvement by cancer in this precise site (in the "aorto-pulmonary recess") was associated with a somewhat more favorable prognosis for surgical cure than was lymph node involvement elsewhere in the mediastinum.[1] Still, the odds against Alfredo's survival had been long, almost remote.

RAY SULLIVAN. MARCH 1968.

In 1968, Dr. Bill Hunter still was one of the junior faculty members, scheduled as a result to take his turn at attending duties on the thoracic surgery service at the Veterans' Administration Hospital in West Roxbury. Mostly, this involved supervising the skilled and highly capable senior residents, discussing and approving their consultations on other services, their plans for each of their own patients, and the like, also scrubbing with them in the operating room on major and serious cases. He made informal rounds with the residents and the students at least once a week, to see all patients on the service, and usually on Wednesday afternoon attended the thoracic surgery outpatient clinic to see any new patients who might need to be admitted.

On this particular Wednesday the resident asked him to see a new patient, an employee of the hospital who currently worked as a maintenance supervisor. Ray Sullivan was forty-six years old, lived in Dedham, had smoked since his teens. For a couple of months he had been aware of a persistent cough, and the week before had coughed up a little bit of blood. He thought he might have lost a few pounds; otherwise he had remained active and had continued to work full time. He had had no other significant illnesses. His military service had been in North Africa and Italy. The chest x-rays taken in the clinic that day revealed a mass in the right lower lobe, close to the hilum. It gave every appearance of being lung cancer.

Bill Hunter and the resident, Dr. Jim Peabody, talked to Ray at length. He should be admitted to the hospital for biopsy and tests, and surgery if that were found to be appropriate. Ray had no private health insurance in force and was willing to be treated at the V.A. Hospital; his admission was scheduled for the beginning of the next week. The tumor could be seen at bronchoscopy, and biopsies were read as showing moderately well differentiated squamous cell carcinoma. Node biopsy in the neck, and the appropriate scans, were unrevealing. The surgery was done by Dr. Peabody, with Bill assisting. Removal of the entire right lung was necessary, but grossly the tumor was entirely contained within the lung, and none of the hilar or mediastinal nodes were involved. Ray's postoperative course was largely uneventful, and he was discharged on the ninth day. He returned to work only three weeks after discharge.

Almost a year later, in February 1969, Ray was readmitted to the hospital with complaints of progressive headaches, lethargy, and confusion, together with increasing weakness of the left side of his body. It appeared certain that he had developed a metastasis in the brain, but the methods for proving or visualizing it were primitive by today's standards; CT scans and magnetic resonance imaging still were far in the future. Cerebral arteriograms (injection of the arteries of the brain so as to visualize them by X-ray) and an isotope brain scan were compatible with the presence of a tumor on the right side. By the best available indications, it appeared to be solitary. The neurosurgery consultants were in favor of immediate operation; Ray and his wife agreed, and so far as could be determined, the tumor was entirely removed. Again Ray tolerated the operation well. He was given no additional treatment of any kind. This time, he was able to return to work after a couple of months and from then on was capable of full activity, with no residual difficulties.

In later years, Bill Hunter heard occasionally that Ray continued to do well; once Bill reviewed his hospital record for inclusion in a paper that he was writing on lung cancer. Later, after he gave up attending duties at the V.A. Hospital, Bill lost touch with Ray and heard no more for a long time. In 1986, he received a note from another doctor, a family practitioner in Rutland, Vermont, asking if the history he had received from Ray was really true. Ray had retired to Vermont after having worked till he was past sixty, and his story had sounded incredible to his new doctor. Ray had remained entirely well for the seventeen years' interval since his second operation; he had quit smoking after the first and never touched a cigarette again. Bill answered the note saying that Ray's story was true enough, also that a couple of similar patients were being followed at the John C. Warren Memorial, while additional long-surviving patients had been recorded from other medical centers.[2]

How could Ray have achieved such spectacularly long survival after treatment? Metastasis, or spread, of lung cancer to the brain ordinarily is a hopeless disaster. Beth Anderson and Harold Carson had been so afflicted; although Harold had received palliative benefit from radiation treatment, there never had been any possibility of cure for either of them. Beth was found initially to have spread of the disease elsewhere besides the brain, while in Harold's case there had been multiple lesions in the brain. In a very few cases, a solitary brain metastasis may accompany a relatively small tumor in the lung, and both may be cleanly removable by surgery. Such treatment can result in significant benefit for at least some, and in cure for a few. Some patients have undergone craniotomy or removal of the brain lesion first, while some like Ray have developed signs of the brain metastasis late, after removal of the lung tumor. Success apparently is possible either way, provided that the patients have been studied carefully to be sure that there is no other spread and therefore that such an aggressive approach is justified.

GERALDINE ROBERTS. JUNE 1977.

Geraldine and her husband had moved to the Boston area from Hartford only recently. He worked for the Prudential Insurance Company, and this had been a routine transfer. They had not yet found a new family doctor or made many of the other arrangements for newcomers. Since the move, Geraldine had felt a nagging pain in her back, located on both sides just below the points of the shoulder blades; it was not disabling, but it was persistent and worried her a good deal. A neighbor suggested her own physician, who maintained his office for family practice not far away, and Geraldine made an appointment to see him.

The doctor found Geraldine to be tense and worried. She was forty-five, had undergone an appendectomy in childhood, had intermittent pelvic discomfort for ten or twelve years which her former physician had attributed to endometriosis. There had been no other serious illnesses. She took no medications, except for occasional tranquilizers. She had been a smoker since her teens, two packs a day over the last few years which she attributed to various worries and tensions. She had some morning cough without any sputum, and had noted somewhat increased shortness of breath with exertion. There had been a gradual weight loss of as much as eight to ten pounds over the past couple of years. Otherwise, the doctor could note no abnormal signs. He had her go for a chest X-ray and films of the spine; the latter were not abnormal, but the chest film showed a poorly defined two-centimeter density in the right upper lobe. The last chest X-rays from Hartford were obtained for comparison; they were dated two and a half years previously and showed no abnormality. It seemed unlikely that the spot in her lung could be related to her complaint of pain, since the pain was located on both sides, and considerably lower down than the level of the spot. Probably the pain had represented some sort of back strain, but the spot in the lung was a worry for two reasons: first, it was new within the past two years or so; and, second, she had been a long-time smoker. The physician advised consultation with a thoracic surgeon, and got her an appointment to see Dr. Bill Hunter.

Bill Hunter reviewed the recent films plus the old ones from Hartford, and talked to her and her husband at length. The probabilities were heavily in favor of the spot being a cancer, so much so that there would be little reason to go through the various biopsy procedures beforehand. If needle or other biopsies showed cancer, the right upper lobe would have to be removed; if they did not, the spot could not be disregarded and it would have to be removed in any case to settle the question. To disregard the spot, or to observe it over a period of time, would be to subject her to unwarranted additional risk. Geraldine and her husband were worried about the problem and asked Bill to proceed.

In the hospital, an isotope bone scan and several additional bone X-rays were unrevealing. The pain of which she had complained originally had largely subsided. Her electrocardiogram was normal, and tests of her breathing were satisfactory. At the operation, the lump could be felt within the right upper lobe, close to the surface of the lung; a biopsy and frozen section confirmed that it was cancer, and a right upper lobectomy was done. Geraldine was young and tolerated the operation well, but there was a relatively prolonged air leak from her chest tubes, and even after they had been removed, another tube had to be placed because of partial collapse of the two remaining lobes. She could not be discharged from the hospital until the sixteenth day after the operation. The final pathologist's report stated that the tumor was a poorly differentiated adenocarcinoma, showing visible spread in the lymphatic channels within the lobe; this was regarded as an ominous prognostic sign but nothing much could be done to change it.

After the first few postoperative visits to Dr. Hunter's office, Geraldine was doing well without any particular complaints. Her breathing was fairly good, and for a few months she had a slight dry cough which later subsided. She had quit smoking for good. About a year after the operation, she was worried by a return of the pain in her back, between the shoulder blades. New X-rays, a new bone scan, and evaluation by other consultants could find no particular cause for it. Eventually the problem seemed to resolve itself. She continued to return to Bill's office every six months for a follow-up examination and new chest X-rays, always without abnormal findings. Bill saw her last at six years after the operation. It was agreed that she could return to her own physician from that time on, but should continue to have an X-ray once a year for a few more years and could return to see Bill in case of any problem or question.

Good fortune had been a factor in Geraldine's long survival. She had developed a troublesome unrelated symptom, pain in the back, which led her to see a physician even though it had no especial link to the small cancer that was found. Most early and curable lung cancers are discovered incidentally, before they are causing symptoms, and usually on an X-ray taken for some other reason. The pathologist's finding of tumor cells beginning to spread within the lymphatic channels is a likely predictor of poor result and short survival; nonetheless, she had done well. No single sign necessarily proves that the patient's outlook is hopeless, unless it is the finding of spread to multiple distant sites, or multiple brain lesions.

CHARLES MORAN. MAY 1974.

Charles Moran was scheduled for admission to Newton-Wellesley Hospital on Sunday for repair of an inguinal hernia, a "rupture" in the groin; he had gone in on the previous Wednesday afternoon to have his preadmission cardiogram, chest X-ray, and drawing of blood specimens. On Thursday afternoon his doctor's office called to say that his chest X-ray had been reported as abnormal. Since the operation was elective and not urgent, his admission to the hospital would have to be canceled at least until this new problem had been resolved. Could he come in to the office the next afternoon to talk with Dr. Wilder about it?

Dr. George Wilder was a general surgeon who practiced in the west suburban area; he had made a point of looking at Charles's films himself after having been notified that they were abnormal. There was a large mass in the left lung, about seven centimeters in diameter and located near the hilum, almost certainly a cancer of the lung. Dr. Wilder explained the problem to Charles and his wife, saying it was important for him to see a thoracic surgeon. George had known Bill Hunter while he himself had been a resident in surgery and Bill a junior member of the faculty. An appointment was made for Charles to see him early the next week.

Bill found Charles to be a large man, easygoing and friendly. He was sixty and worked as a machine operator. He had been a smoker most of his life, but had quit this past winter during a severe and persistent respiratory infection. Since quitting, his breathing and his appetite had improved; he had gained ten to twelve pounds. He had continued to work full time and insisted that he felt well, but on close questioning admitted that he had coughed up some tiny flecks of blood during the past few weeks. A slight change in the breath sounds could be heard over his left lung. There were no signs of tumor spread. The hernia that originally had led to all these questions was causing him occasional discomfort, no real pain or other problems. He was willing to be admitted to the hospital for diagnosis and treatment.

At bronchoscopy, Bill could not visualize the tumor itself, but could see distortion of the bronchi on the left as though from external pressure. Washings were reported as positive for malignant cells, the precise cell type not being entirely clear. Mediastinoscopy done at the same time was without abnormal findings. Isotope scans of the liver and brain were called normal; Charles had had no pain or soreness in the bones, and a bone scan was omitted. His breathing tests appeared marginal since removal of the whole lung would probably be necessary, but Bill had Charles climb stairs with him and found that he could go up five flights at a steady walk. By Bill's personal rule of thumb, this level of performance should allow a patient to survive pneumonectomy without severe disability. Bill sat down with Charles and his wife, as he tried to do with all patients, to advise that he undergo surgery and to answer their questions and discuss with them the limitations of surgical treatment and its potential dangers. Charles would not hear any discussion of the dangers, or the possibilities of failure; he said twice, "Doctor, I'm in your hands. I want you to do what is necessary, and I'm not going to worry about any risks or other details." It did not help for Bill to point out that he was obligated to obtain informed consent from patients, to make sure that they and their families understood what was being discussed, that they agreed with the plan, and that any questions had been answered. But Charles preferred to agree without discussion, and signed the permit for the operation without glancing at the paragraphs of fine print.

At the operation, the tumor was found as a large mass, close to the hilum, and removal of the whole lung was necessary. No signs of spread could be seen. Charles's recovery was uneventful, untroubled by worries or depression. He was back on his feet within a few days and resumed ambulation, although bothered somewhat by shortness of breath. The pathologist's report described the tumor as moderately well differentiated squamous cell carcinoma; the lines of resection were clear, and there was no involvement of lymph nodes. Plainly, no additional treatment was warranted.

At his first office visit, two weeks after discharge from the hospital, Charles was cheerful and said that he was doing well. His appetite was good, and the soreness from the operation practically gone. He admitted that his breathing was shorter, but he was adjusting his level of activity to cope with it. From that time on, Bill saw him for routine follow-up visits every six months. Five years after the operation, Charles was well and his chest X-rays were unchanged, but his blood pressure was somewhat high. Since he had never had a family doctor, Bill advised that he get one to look after his blood pressure and the other problems of increasing age. Bill had to readmit him to the hospital once for treatment of pneumonia in the other lung, nine years after the operation, but did not see him again after that. Bill learned later from Charles's own doctor that he was alive and reasonably well in 1988, fourteen years after the operation. He was then aged seventy-four. He had gotten by without ever having the original hernia repaired.

Again, Charles's cancer had been discovered incidentally, on X-rays done for another reason, so that his situation was potentially more favorable than most. It would not be right to say that the tumor had caused him no symptoms, since he had coughed up a few flecks of blood during the weeks before the tumor was discovered. It cannot be said, either, that his attitude or mental state were responsible for his long survival after surgery; the mutation of the tumor cells' DNA is not susceptible to control by positive thinking, whatever we may have read in popular journals. Another factor was in his favor, that the tumor was a squamous cell carcinoma which, although large, had shown little tendency to spread. Squamous cell carcinomas do not by any means all behave in this way, but the lung cancers which are found to be still localized are most often of this type. How long had it been present before discovery? Without having frequent old X-rays available, there is no way to tell, but some similar lung cancers have been observed to have grown slowly over a number of years.[3]

EVA LOPRESTI. JANUARY 1977.

Early in December, Eva had developed a cough with fever, and pain in the left side of her chest especially when coughing or breathing deeply. She had gone to see her physician, Dr. Michel LeBeau, who had listened to her chest, then sent her for an X-ray which revealed a small area of streaky shadows extending from the hilum of the left lung out to the chest wall in the left upper lobe. The radiologist read these changes as being consistent with pneumonia. Dr. LeBeau had given her a prescription for an antibiotic capsule to be taken four times a day and advised her to stay home from work and rest. Her fever and the chest pain declined in a few days, but the dry, racking cough persisted. After a month at home, she had returned to see him and the chest X-ray was repeated; this film showed no improvement over the one in December, and the streaky shadows were still present. Her problem, whatever it might be, was not so simple, and her doctor saw that it would have to be looked into more carefully.

Eva was only forty, had two children in the fifth and eighth grades. She worked as a product inspector at a machine tool factory in Greenfield, Massachusetts. Her husband was a bus driver and mechanic for the Greenfield school system. She had not had any serious illnesses but had smoked since the age of fifteen. She was slight in build, thin, but did not think she had lost any weight in the last month or two. There were no other symptoms, no change in her appetite, no headaches, no new aches or pains. The persistence of her cough and of the shadows in her lung worried Dr. LeBeau; if it were due only to a small area of pneumonia, it should have cleared before now. He advised that she go to Boston for consultation, and made an appointment for her to see Dr. Hunter. She was to take along both sets of X-rays.

Bill Hunter listened to her story, could get no particular new information about her symptoms, and could find no abnormalities on examination. The X-ray films, dated about a month apart, showed no mass or lump, but the streaky density extending out from the left hilum gave the appearance of atelectasis of the anterior segment of the left upper lobe, one segment out of five in the lobe. The density had persisted without improvement in spite of her treatment with antibiotics, and she had been a long-time smoker. His concern would have to be for the possibility of lung cancer. He advised admission to the hospital as soon as it would be convenient for her. She had been off work for a month already and was willing to be admitted that weekend.

Bill reflected that atelectasis of a lobe or segment was a convenient marker for the surgeon at bronchoscopy, because it told him precisely where to look for the tumor, and that the tumor would be visible within reach of the scope. The new slim, flexible fiberoptic bronchoscopes had greatly improved the possibilities of this examination. Bill scheduled bronchoscopy and mediastinoscopy for the morning after Eva was admitted. Through the scope he could identify the anterior segment bronchus precisely, and saw that its orifice was plugged by a rounded, fleshy growth, as expected. A tiny biopsy of this tissue was reported later as showing well differentiated squamous cell carcinoma. Mediastinoscopy was unrevealing, without any abnormal nodes, and the routine scans also showed no abnormalities. Eva was young for a patient with lung cancer. Her electrocardiogram was normal, and the tests of her breathing were satisfactory. Bill discussed the problem with Eva and her husband and advised surgical removal. They were doubtful at first and unwilling to agree. Bill felt that in this situation, he was obligated to apply some pressure on them; she was young, there was proof that her trouble was due to cancer, and by all indications, the cancer was small and in an early stage. Eventually they agreed, and the procedure was scheduled.

At the operation, the anterior segment of the upper lobe was found to be densely contracted by atelectasis and chronic infection. There were some adhesions between this area and the chest wall, but the remainder of the lung was clear. The upper lobe was removed, and after it was cut for closer examination, the little plug of tumor in the anterior segment bronchus could be seen once more. It was less than one centimeter in diameter, about three-tenths of an inch, and arose from one side of the segmental bronchus. Later, the pathologist's report confirmed that the tumor was a squamous cell carcinoma; none of eleven lymph nodes in the specimen were involved. Eva's recovery was uneventful, and she was discharged from the hospital on the sixth day.

She returned for a follow-up visit two weeks after discharge, doing well and with the cough almost gone. Soreness from the operation had practically disappeared, her appetite was good, and she was increasing her activity at home. Because of the distance to Boston, she asked if she could go back to Dr. LeBeau for follow-up and Bill agreed. He tried his best to warn her against continued smoking, but she declined to make any promises. Thereafter, she did not return. Much later, Bill received a note from Dr. LeBeau saying that she had passed five years since the operation and remained well; he did not say whether she had quit smoking.

Once again, to have any reasonable chance of cure in lung cancer, medicine has no substitute for early diagnosis and treatment. The few slowly-growing and late-spreading cancers which have grown to considerable size before discovery, as Charles Moran's had done, are only minor exceptions to the rule; they are so rare that their inclusion does not significantly affect cure rates or median survival of all patients. In Eva LoPresti's case, the tumor was tiny, less than a centimeter in diameter, had not spread to any of the nodes, and was well-differentiated squamous cell carcinoma in type. Plainly, her prognosis would be good after surgical removal of the tumor. But how was her tumor discovered in such an early stage? She was fortunate that the tiny cancer had produced symptoms indirectly; the persistent cough and fever had been caused by infection beyond an obstruction in the bronchus, therefore they were only secondarily due to the tumor. Located anywhere else than at the orifice of a segmental bronchus, the tumor would have caused no symptoms at this early stage, and in all probability Eva would not have seen her physician until more serious symptoms had developed.

Thirteen

FACTORS OF CURABILITY

You want to lead
My reason blindfold like a hamper'd lion,
Check'd of his noble vigor—then, when baited
Down to obedient tameness, make it couch
And show strange tricks which you call signs of faith.

—Thomas Otway, *Venice Preserved* (1682)

WHAT IS CURE?

When an operation is completed, and the patient's condition is stable enough, the surgeon's first obligation is to speak with the patient's family and inform them of the entire situation. Naturally, the family always has questions; if the operation has been for cancer, they invariably ask, "Doctor, did you get it all?" Dr. Bill Hunter, for one, has always found this question impossible to answer in the family's terms. The answer they want to hear is an unequivocal yes. Can the surgeon, aware of human limitations as well as of the uncertainties inherent in lung cancer treatment, ever answer with such confidence? Bill is aware that many surgeons do answer in just that way, never mind the prospects for the future. He finds that if he equivocates even slightly in answering the question, if he explains that the surgeon is unable to see or identify microscopic tumor spread, that he removed all that could be seen, but that only time can tell whether he "got it all," the relatives' faces fall and they are likely to be bitterly disappointed. Most of them believe, in fact, that they are being told the patient has not been cured and cannot be. Bill speaks gently but in the plainest of terms when the news is bad, when the family has to understand that there is no possibility of cure, because they will have to make their plans accordingly. But cure is never assured under the best of circumstances. Knowing that recurrence of the disease is always possible, at an unpredictable time, Bill is unable to answer the question with a simple clear affirmative while still retaining any regard for the truth. There are too many uncertainties involved.

Of 100 consecutive patients at the time of first diagnosis of lung cancer, at least 55 will have inoperable disease; that is, their disease is spreading and cannot be removed, or they would be unable to tolerate the surgery. Of the remaining 45 or so, 10 to 15 are found at the operation to have disease unsuited to curative resection, meaning that there is involvement of nearby structures that cannot be spared, so that clean removal is not possible. Thirty to 35, at best, can undergo resection "for cure"; the phrase does not mean that they will be cured, only that the surgeon was able to remove all the grossly visible tumor.

Patients in this last group, having had surgery with intent to cure, still face an uncertain future. Of those who have undergone pneumonectomy, removal of an entire lung, 15 to 20 percent will be alive five years later, while those who have undergone lobectomy do somewhat better; 30 to 35 percent will survive at least five years. It may seem paradoxical that the lesser operation has the better cure rate. The main factor controlling long survival is not the extent of the operation itself but the stage of disease at the time of treatment. If the patient's cancer is a large mass close to the hilum, which cannot be removed except by removal of the entire lung, the patient's chance of survival will be poorer than if the cancer is a small nodule in the periphery of the lung, cleanly removable by lobectomy or even by segmental resection. (Few patients should undergo removal of lung cancer by less than lobectomy.) Finally, of the 100 original patients, no more than 8 or 9 will remain alive after 5 years. This figure, known as the Salvage Rate, is the final index to effectiveness of treatment. Occasionally one sees a higher figure quoted, in the range of 12 to 14 percent, but these series have included the so-called bronchial adenomas, a group of low-grade malignancies that are for the most part curable. Bronchial adenomas bear no relation to smoking, their behavior is not comparable to that of true lung cancer, and their inclusion in a survey of treatment results serves only to make the results look better than they really are.

Survival without recurrence for five years after treatment of lung cancer is a fairly secure indication that the disease has been eradicated, or "cured." (Some other malignancies, such as breast cancer, may recur as late as twenty years or even more after treatment, so that five year follow-up is not enough.) Most relapses of lung cancer occur within two to three years, and recurrence after that time is rare, so that "disease-free" survival for three years is almost as favorable as for five. It is possible, though, for a second lung cancer to develop later even if the first cancer has been cured. The same causative factor has been at work elsewhere in the lung.

Within this generally gloomy picture are a few brighter spots, principally concerning those patients whose cancers are discovered in an early stage. I have mentioned occult carcinomas, defining them as not visible on the chest X-ray but identified by positive sputum cytology, the finding of malignant cells in the sputum. Such cancers are almost always squamous cell in type. Only a few institutions have accumulated much experience with occult carcinomas, but they have found that most can eventually be localized by careful, systematic fiberoptic bronchoscopy, brushing from each segmental bronchus, and repeating the examination every two to three months if necessary. If reliably localized to a given segment or lobe, and removed surgically, such tumors are almost all curable. Radiation therapy in the same situation has been a disappointment, failing to show curative effect. Unfortunately, lung cancer rarely is discovered in the occult stage.

Early disease, in any form, tends to be associated with better prognosis than the overall figures would suggest. The earliest stage-group of cancers identifiable by X-ray would be classed as having: (1) diameter of 3 centimeters (about one and one-fifth inches) or less; (2) peripheral location, so that they are seen on the X-ray to be surrounded by clear lung; and (3) no spread either to lymph nodes or distant sites. (These are classed as T1 N0 M0 in the TNM system). Approximately 80 percent of such patients have remained well five years after surgical removal,[1] a figure so high that it would be almost impossible for a study of adjuvant treatment to show significant added benefit to survival. As disease stage progresses beyond this highly select group, survival rates decline sharply.

Patients with cancers in the form of asymptomatic peripheral coin lesions, promptly removed by surgery, have a 40 to 50 percent probability of five-year survival. This figure is dependent on their having experienced no symptoms. Observation of such cancers by periodic X-rays until they are seen to enlarge can only be detrimental, since two studies have found that successive increments in tumor diameter of one centimeter, or one and a half centimeters, are associated with declining chances of five year survival.[2]

In approximate order of importance, factors responsible for declining probability of long survival include tumor size larger than three centimeters diameter; spread to hilar lymph nodes; spread to mediastinal lymph nodes; tumor invasion of the chest wall, or of the mediastinum to a limited degree. Factors which practically eliminate any chance of cure are spread to lymph nodes in the neck, or in the opposite side of the mediastinum; invasion of mediastinal structures which cannot be removed, such as the great vessels, the trachea, the left or right atrium, or the bony vertebrae; and spread to distant sites, with only the barest few possible exceptions as noted. Added to these should be any factors interfering with the patient's ability to tolerate the operation and survive, which include heart disease, pulmonary insufficiency, advanced weight loss, weakness or disability, and problems of blood clotting.

CAN THE ODDS BE IMPROVED?

Having noted that 30 to 35 of the 100 original patients can undergo surgery with the hope of cure, but that only 8 or 9 out of the hundred will survive for 5 years, we might ask: What has happened to the remainder, who do not survive? Almost all have developed recurrence of the disease, either within the chest or at some distant site. Grossly identifiable recurrence of lung cancer after treatment is—with rare exception—by definition incurable. Survival of these patients could be improved, in theory, if some method were available to wipe out the invisible spreading cancer cells that may remain after surgery, since at this time their number should be at its lowest. Chemotherapy might do so, given as a supplement to surgical treatment, and was the object of many high hopes in the past. Within the limits of this discussion, chemotherapy has not lived up to its promise. No randomized, prospective study of adjuvant chemotherapy has found that it increases cure rates in non-small-cell carcinoma of the lung. Possibly some of the newer regimens based on cisplatin may soon begin to show such a difference. Any real benefit would be a great thing since it would appear as an increase in the proportion of cures. Toxicity from treatment would surely be more acceptable if it offered an increased measure of hope.

Great enthusiasm arose in the past for immunotherapy, the concept that the host's immune system can be sensitized, or stimulated, to eradicate a small remaining burden of cancer cells. Certain cancers of small animals, mice and rats, could be treated successfully and even cured, but unfortunately those tumors were not valid models of spontaneous cancer, and the results were bogus. So far at least, the glowing prospects for immunotherapy's effectiveness against human lung cancer have remained unproved; no positive findings have ever been independently confirmed. A different aspect of the immune system, which I discuss in the last chapter, may hold promise.

DOES THE PATIENT "BATTLE" HIS CANCER?

Popular wisdom about cancer has created an image of the indomitable patient, who will not accept a fatal illness and wages a valiant struggle to overcome it. Then if he has been cured, the patient becomes a hero who has "beaten" his disease. The late John Wayne (1907–1979), possibly America's favorite movie actor, announced to the press that he was "going to lick the Big C" when he was found in 1964 to have lung cancer. (He was fifty-seven at the time, had smoked on screen and off since his teens.) Indeed he did, if one chooses not to remember that he underwent a completely successful resection, at which time the cancer was found to be localized. He survived for fifteen years after surgery, but died in 1979 of cancer of the colon; the new tumor was more advanced when discovered than the first had been.

Dr. Bill Hunter remembers the family of a young patient with lung cancer, admitted to the hospital in a desperate state without any possibility of recovery. As things grew worse, some of his family would growl through gritted teeth, "Heeza fighter! Heez gonna lick it!" He may indeed have been a fighter, and courageous—but none of those things mattered now. Tragically, this view forgets that when the patient dies we have to presume that he or she failed to "fight" properly. It follows that he or she must have been a weakling, or a poltroon. The words are not spoken aloud, but the patient is said to have "lost a long battle with cancer." The idea is thoroughly ingrained into the collective American consciousness, yet it is a cruel fallacy. Who would like to find himself in the condition of Beth Anderson, say, or of Andy Cunningham, at the time of first diagnosis? Could you, or anyone, make up your mind to "lick it," and proceed to do so? As you grew weaker and thinner, and knew in your heart you were dying, could you tolerate the thought of being a coward, unwilling to "fight" the disease successfully?

Many readers will not accept that "fighting" cancer is a delusion, and even some physicians are inclined to agree. A celebrated book, the first author of which is an M.D. from California, has undertaken to coach the cancer patient through the mental attitudes and disciplines that are promised to overcome his cancer.[3] The Simonton treatment, among other things, prescribes daily sessions of relaxation and cultivation of favorable mental imagery, during which the subject is to visualize his white blood cells (strong and purposeful) destroying the cancer cells (weak and confused). The treatment advocates a way of thinking, not as an end in itself, but literally as a means of defeating the disease.

Such talk strikes a responsive chord in the minds of many cancer patients, even those who are intelligent and well-informed. Surely the attraction is that the patient seems to be offered a choice, the right to control his own treatment. But when the treatment fails, responsibility for failure is transferred to the patient, because he did not participate strongly enough or enthusiastically enough. The practitioner is absolved of responsibility, because it was not his negligence or error but the patient's lack of enthusiasm that caused a poor result. A surgeon writing of his experience as a patient with incurable lung cancer has told of the comfort he derived from the Simonton program of therapeutic meditation and mental imagery.[4] Yet he died in December 1985, a year after publication of his personal account.[5] We have no information on what he thought of the power of mind over body near the end.

The cancer clinic staff at a university medical center has studied a group of their patients to try to determine what effect, if any, the patient's mental and psychological state might have upon the course of their disease.[6] A total of 204 patients with unresectable cancer of various types were followed to determine their length of survival. Another 155 patients who had undergone successful surgical treatment for localized melanoma, or for intermediate-stage breast cancer, were followed to determine their time to first relapse. All were evaluated at the beginning of treatment by a self-reporting questionnaire, plus personal interviews. Both evaluations sought to determine the patients' psychological state according to seven variables which previously had been reported to have an effect on survival:

1. Social ties and marital history.
2. Job satisfaction.
3. Use or non-use of mind-altering drugs.
4. General life evaluation, and satisfaction.
5. Subjective view of health in adult life.
6. Degree of feelings of helplessness, hopelessness.
7. Perception of adjustment required to cope with the new diagnosis of cancer.

The study could find no correlations between psychosocial factors and the patients' survival, or time until recurrence. A thoughtful editorial in the same issue of the journal concluded: "It is time to acknowledge that our belief in disease as a direct reflection of mental state is largely folklore. Furthermore, the corollary view of sickness and death as a personal failure is a particularly unfortunate form of blaming the victim. At a time when patients are already burdened by disease, they should not be further burdened by having to accept responsibility for the outcome."[7]

SPONTANEOUS REGRESSION

I cannot close this chapter without reference to a bizarre aspect of cancer, potentially hopeful but one over which we have no control. Proof of cancer diagnosis by microscopic examination of tissue, as from a biopsy, has been available since the nineteenth century. Since the latter part of the century, at least, occasional instances have been recorded of the disappearance of cancer without treatment, or with inadequate treatment. Termed "spontaneous regression," such occurrences naturally have excited tremendous interest because they seemed to suggest that cancer may in fact be vulnerable. Several reviews have looked for common factors, or underlying similarities between cases, unfortunately without much success. Proven and well-documented cases of spontaneous regression are exceedingly rare. The largest collective review of the subject recorded complete or partial regression of many different types of cancer, but of only one case of lung cancer.[8] This patient had undergone thoracotomy at which time the tumor had been found unresectable, but during a six months' period after the operation the remaining tumor was seen by X-ray to diminish in size. The patient remained alive more than five years after surgery, at which time metastatic lesions had appeared in bone. No further information about the patient's survival has been published since. This case would have to be regarded as an instance of partial regression, not complete regression or cure.

A more striking example was reported in 1964. The patient, a young man in his late thirties, also had undergone thoracotomy with the finding that the disease could not be removed.[9] Following surgery, he was given radiation therapy to that side of the chest, but in a dose thought entirely insufficient to cause the changes that followed. After his recovery from treatment he resorted to hard physical labor on a farm, believing that he himself could aid the struggle against his disease. Subsequent chest films showed gradual clearing of the tumor densities in his lung, while he remained in robust good health. (It is recorded that he continued to smoke.) His amazing recovery was the subject of a story in the Seattle *Times* in 1971, twelve years after his unsuccessful operation.[10]

Bill Hunter had been intrigued by this last report, but had no cause to doubt it; soon after the end of his residency training he had seen another case just as dramatic. Bill had been at the weekly thoracic surgery outpatient clinic in the V.A. hospital when a patient returned for his routine annual follow-up visit, now just over five years since he had undergone surgery. Bill noted with astonishment that his entire right lung had been removed, with the pathologic diagnosis of undifferentiated small-cell carcinoma; also that the surgeon's note described numerous large mediastinal lymph nodes involved by the tumor, the largest "the size of a fist," which were removed as well as possible. No chemotherapy regimens for small-cell carcinoma of the lung existed at that time, and the patient had received no other treatment. An X-ray film dated about eighteen months after the surgery showed a patch of infiltrate in the opposite lung, thought to have represented pneumonia. On subsequent films this had cleared and no further abnormalities could be seen. The attending surgeon whose name was on the operative note had moved away about a year later and was in practice with a large private clinic on the West Coast.

Such a chronology would sound incredible in any type of lung cancer, most of all in small-cell carcinoma. We think of cancer as a disease of relentless progression, but it is clear that regression can occur, however rarely, and even to the extent of a spontaneous cure. A couple of explanations are not beyond scientific possibility: first, that a genetic change in the tumor cells may reverse the malignant phenotype, in the direction of cell differentiation and stability. This is known to occur occasionally in cases of a childhood malignancy called neuroblastoma. Second, many of the older reports of spontaneous regression described it as occurring during or after certain infections which were associated with a high fever, particularly scarlet fever and erysipelas, infections which have been almost unknown since the advent of penicillin. The immune system and its responses are not yet thoroughly understood; some investigators believe that under special or unusual circumstances, a febrile illness may activate "killer cells" sufficiently that a cancer may be eradicated. The difficulty so far is that the biologic or chemical controls to induce such an activation remain largely out of our grasp. Fever alone is not sufficient.

The two patients reported as having shown spontaneous regression of lung cancer were said to have had febrile periods during recovery from operation.[11] All patients are likely to have fever for at least a few days in the postoperative period; did these have more than most? Probably not, at least so far as can be determined from the brief reports. Bill Hunter studied the hospital record of the patient he saw in the V.A. clinic, but there had been no unusually high or prolonged fever. Could there have been high or prolonged fever during the supposed episode of pneumonia, eighteen months after the operation? The man had not been admitted to the hospital, and no other records existed. Eighteen months after his operation, at which time only incomplete removal of the tumor had been possible, a patient with small-cell carcinoma of the lung ordinarily would long since have died. An immune reaction leading to spontaneous regression, if there had been one, must have occurred earlier. As usual, the records provided no easy answer.

Fourteen

THE VARIANT: SMALL-CELL CARCINOMA

You may think, passer-by, that Fate
Is a pit-fall outside of yourself,
Around which you may walk by the use of foresight
And wisdom. . . . But pass on into life:
In time you shall see Fate approach you
In the shape of your own image in the mirror;
Or you shall sit alone by your own hearth,
And suddenly the chair by you shall hold a guest,
And you shall know that guest,
And read the authentic message of his eyes.

—Edgar Lee Masters, "Lyman King," *Spoon River Anthology* (1914)

CAROLINE DEUTSCH. JANUARY 1975.

Caroline had stayed home from work for three days and was feeling no better. She did not have a family doctor, so went to the emergency room at the John C. Warren Memorial to be seen. She had been head nurse on the evening shift there for some years, on one of the surgical floors; it was the place she knew best. Several years before, she had been admitted for gall bladder surgery and had developed great respect for her surgeon, Dr. James Winthrop. She gave his name as her choice when she was seen at the emergency room.

Dr. Winthrop was free and came down to see her before she was admitted. Caroline was fifty-four, had had no serious illnesses except for the gallbladder trouble. Her husband stayed at home, partially disabled by arthritis. She had worked at the John C. Warren for almost twenty years now. For the past two to three weeks she had felt tired, easily fatigued, and for the last four days had noted vague abdominal distress but no cramps or nausea. Her appetite had been poor for the last few days; she was not sure whether she had lost any weight. She had smoked since age eighteen and was aware that her cough had been more persistent lately. Dr. Winthrop noted on examination that her liver was enlarged, somewhat lumpy in outline, and moderately tender to pressure. Plainly, she needed to be in the hospital for diagnostic studies. He arranged for her to have X-rays of the chest and abdomen during admission, plus a liver scan the next morning.

The chest films demonstrated a mass in the right upper lobe, also a large irregular mediastinal density indicative of extensive node involvement. The liver scan revealed an enlarged liver with numerous lucent areas suggesting multiple metastatic lesions. Metastatic from where? The densities in her lung and mediastinum, plus her long smoking history, pointed to lung cancer as the first probability. A CT study of the chest generally confirmed these findings. Already the disease was shockingly extensive. Jim Winthrop was a general surgeon and did not deal with lung cancer; he asked Bill Hunter for consultation and assistance.

Bill too had known Caroline, from her long association with the hospital, and talked with her at length about the problem. He asked permission to schedule her for bronchoscopy and mediastinoscopy the next morning, with the aim of establishing a diagnosis. He could see nothing abnormal at bronchoscopy but was not surprised since the mass was relatively far out in the lung; at mediastinoscopy there was a conglomerate mass of enlarged lymph nodes in the upper mediastinum, from which he took biopsies. The pathologist's report stated that nodes were replaced by undifferentiated small-cell carcinoma.

Surgical treatment was out of the question for two reasons: because of widespread metastatic disease, but also because of the unfavorable cell type. Then as now, small-cell carcinoma was regarded as essentially incurable by surgery because of its rapid growth and early spread; in fact until about two years before, no treatment had seemed to make any difference. One of the young oncologists at the Lowell-Eliot Cancer Institute had recently returned from a fellowship at Bethesda, Maryland, eager to put to work the new interest in combined modality treatment for small-cell carcinoma of the lung. Bill already had referred a couple of patients to him and had been impressed by their responses to chemotherapy. Careful staging by numerous studies was required before treatment could begin. Caroline had to undergo CT studies of the brain and the abdomen, a bone scan in the Nuclear Medicine Department (a liver scan had already been done), and biopsies of the bone marrow through a needle, from the upper edge of the hip bone. Bone marrow biopsies were positive for tumor cells, so that, in all, the disease was known to have spread to mediastinal nodes, liver, and the bone marrow. Dr. D'Silva, the oncologist, had to ask Caroline to sign several extra permission forms for the treatment, which still was experimental.

The treatment program began with chemotherapy: cyclophosphamide, vincristine, and lomustine (at that time it was called CCNU, chloroethyl-cyclohexyl-nitrosourea); the combination was known among the oncology fellows as the CCV regimen. Caroline had received pretreatment medication intended to minimize the nausea and vomiting caused by these drugs, and she tolerated the first course fairly well. She was discharged from the hospital after one day's rest, with arrangements to return weekly for blood counts. Three weeks later, showing good recovery, she received additional doses of cyclophosphamide and vincristine. Lomustine was omitted from the alternate-dose schedule because of its more delayed toxicity, requiring a longer recovery period. Beginning at six weeks after the first dose, there was a short period off chemotherapy to allow for radiation treatments to the primary tumor, the mediastinal mass, and the brain. These were given over a period of two weeks, to a dose level of what still were called 2400 rads, and on the following week chemotherapy was resumed without further interruptions. Dr. D'Silva had explained to Caroline that her hair would begin to fall out from the chemotherapy, more or less completely after the radiation treatments to the brain, but that it might begin to regrow to some degree later on. Like most patients, she had had a wig made beforehand. The treatment program took precedence over everything else in her living schedule, and she had given up her job. She always needed a couple of days to recover from the effects of the drugs, every three weeks, but afterward had only to go in to the clinic once a week for blood counts and a brief check.

By two months after the radiation treatments, she had entered complete remission; her chest X-ray now was clear, and a follow-up liver scan no longer showed any evidence of metastases. Her abdominal distress had long since disappeared. She tired easily and did not feel in robust health, but much of that could be blamed on the continuing treatments. Great promise was held out to her for future improvement after the treatments could be discontinued. Summer and fall went by with unchanging routine. Bill Hunter happened one day to be on the surgical floor where Caroline had worked, when the head nurse of the day shift told him that she had been to visit Caroline at home. Her reaction generally had been one of revulsion; she vowed that she herself would never agree to undergo "chemo" and have to live like that. Caroline herself was happy to remain alive. To Bill Hunter, it was plain that she could not have survived more than three or four weeks from the time of her admission in January without the new treatment program.

By October, Caroline was feeling weaker and beginning to lose weight. Her appetite had deteriorated and there were increasingly painful areas in her bones. Dr. D'Silva found that the metastases in her liver had appeared again, together with new ones in bone. Having recurred while she still was receiving chemotherapy, these could mean only that the tumor had become resistant to the three drugs. Her treatment program was changed to alternative, or second-line drugs, without much benefit. From then on her condition deteriorated rapidly. She was readmitted to the hospital in a terminal state and died in December 1975, eleven months after diagnosis of her cancer.

Had the severe and protracted treatment been worthwhile? Beyond any doubt, it had prolonged her survival, probably by nine or ten months. Was that extra time useful and rewarding to her? Her friend, the other head nurse, did not think so, but in Caroline's mind there had been no doubt. Once begun, there had been no escape from this kind of treatment; it is not given in a day and then it is over, as is surgery for example; it goes on and on until the disease recurs, the patient declines to continue with it further, or the patient passes six months to a year on treatment while remaining in complete remission. Most oncologists will discontinue treatment at such a time in the hope that the disease has been eradicated, and in recognition that chemotherapy is no longer worth its risks after such a period.

AN ESPECIALLY MALIGNANT AFFLICTION

Small-cell carcinoma of the lung was the commonest tumor type of the dreaded *Bergkrankheit* or mountain sickness among uranium and cobalt miners of Central Europe. Today, squamous cell carcinoma shares its menace to persons subjected to radon exposure, but both tumor types retain an exceptionally high association with long-time smoking. As surgical treatment for lung cancer developed gradually in the 1930s and 1940s, small-cell carcinoma was found to be practically incurable; almost always it had spread widely by the time of diagnosis. Yet, it seemed, no other treatment was available. Although the tumor responded well to radiation therapy, widespread disease was unaffected by that method also.

In the late 1950s, the Medical Research Council of Great Britain began a prospective comparative trial of treatment by surgery versus radiation therapy, in patients with localized disease which had been pronounced operable by the thoracic surgical consultants. (At the time, methods for identification of distant disease were relatively crude, so that accurate staging as we now know it was not possible.) Biopsy proof of the disease was required; under the circumstances this could be obtained only through rigid bronchoscopes, a type now largely obsolete. Cooperating hospitals telephoned the center when a patient meeting the criteria had agreed to enter the study, and treatment was assigned by randomization. In all, seventy-three patients were assigned to be treated by radiotherapy, of which four survived more than five years and three for more than ten years. Seventy-one were assigned to be treated by surgery; the only one who survived five years refused surgery and had been treated instead by radiotherapy.[1] The study convinced oncologists everywhere that surgical resection offered no possibility of cure, while radiation therapy offered at least a slight possibility. We see now that patients who might have presented with early disease could not have been admitted to the study, since they would not have had biopsy proof.

Beginning in about 1960, systematic testing of chemotherapeutic drugs against lung cancer in the United States found no benefit from them, except that in small-cell carcinoma the patients' survival was considerably prolonged. A new treatment strategy employed radiation therapy against the bulk of tumor at the primary site and the mediastinal nodes, combined with chemotherapy by several drugs against the widely disseminated component of disease.[2] First reported in 1973, this general scheme has remained the basis for practically all present-day treatment programs. The most "active" or effective drugs include cyclophosphamide (Cytoxan), cisplatin, lomustine, etoposide, doxorubicin (Adriamycin), methotrexate, and the plant alkaloid vincristine. Most treatment programs use three or even four drugs simultaneously, to the maximum dose tolerated by the patient, a more effective arrangement than use of a single drug. Patient response clearly depends on the stage of disease at the beginning of treatment. Careful studies for presence or absence of distant spread are required before treatment, and patients are divided into those with "limited" disease confined to the primary site and the mediastinal nodes, or those with "extensive" disease having spread to distant sites such as brain, liver, bones, or elsewhere.

Today patients with limited disease usually are treated first with one or two cycles of chemotherapy, then given radiation treatment to the disease within the chest, after which chemotherapy is resumed. Radiation treatment generally is given to the whole brain as well, aiming to eradicate any tumor cells lodged there which otherwise would appear later as metastases in the brain. So long as relapse does not occur, chemotherapy may be continued for six months to a year, or to the limit of patient tolerance if that is less. Almost all patients will respond to such a program, and perhaps two-thirds may achieve complete remission so that no identifiable tumor remains, but most of these will suffer relapse eventually. Median patient survival after treatment of limited disease ranges from about twelve to fifteen months, meaning that half the patients survive that long or longer, half for less than that. Patients who remain in complete remission beyond two years after the start of treatment are doing exceptionally well. Perhaps 10 percent of patients treated for limited disease will have eradication of all tumor, in effect a "cure," and may survive beyond five years. (There is no way to identify these patients in advance, and only time can demonstrate a cure.) Patients who abstain from smoking, even if only from the beginning of treatment, have at least some chance of long disease-free survival, while it appears that those who continue to smoke have none.[3]

Patients who have extensive disease do much less well, and are treated differently, usually by chemotherapy alone. It is no help to treat the large primary tumor mass by radiation therapy if the tumor already has spread elsewhere in the body, nor is prophylactic radiation treatment usually given to the brain unless the patient has achieved complete remission. Relatively few patients in this group reach complete remission, and median survival averages perhaps seven to eight months at most. Only a bare few patients, less than 1 percent, are recorded as having achieved long survival without recurrence. Nevertheless it has happened, and while cure is exceedingly rare, it remains a possibility.

In recent years, a few institutions have reexplored the use of surgical removal of the primary tumor, followed by adjuvant chemotherapy in those few patients who are found to have early stage disease at the time of diagnosis.[4] Fewer than 10 percent of patients first presenting with small cell carcinoma have no identifiable spread to the mediastinal nodes, or farther, although there is likely to be microscopic spread in almost all. In such cases, surgical resection of the primary tumor would have the effect of inducing complete remission immediately, while the bone marrow and host defenses still remained untouched. Chemotherapy begun at this time should have its best chance for disease eradication, considering that only a microscopic tumor burden remains. Small numbers of patients treated in this way have shown exceptionally good five-year survival rates.[5] The problem remains that only a few newly diagnosed patients have suitable early-stage and localized disease. The majority of oncologists remain opposed to inclusion of surgery in treatment of small-cell carcinoma.

Without fundamentally new methods of treatment, no prospect of significantly improved survival can be foreseen in this disease. Presently available treatment can induce dramatic remissions, and prolong life, but few patients can be cured.

Fifteen

REASONABLE THERAPEUTIC INTENSITY

We shall go on to the end. . . . We shall defend our
island, whatever the cost may be; we shall fight on the
beaches, we shall fight on the landing-grounds, we
shall fight in the fields and in the streets, we shall
fight in the hills; we shall never surrender.

—Prime Minister Winston Churchill to the
House of Commons, June 4, 1940.

Next to a battle lost, the greatest misery is a battle
gained.

—Arthur Wellesley, Duke of Wellington
(1769–1852)

Consider this problem: You yourself are found to have non-small-cell
cancer of the lung, and undergo lobectomy for its removal. Ten months
after the operation, the disease is found to have recurred in liver and
bones. After suitable studies, treatment by chemotherapy is advised. You
are told plainly of the risks and side effects; also that there will be no
prospect of cure, but only about a 20 percent possibility, at best, of
prolongation of life. Your survival expectancy is estimated at three
months without treatment. Should you agree to undergo treatment at all?
Would you prefer to be treated to the absolute limit of tolerance, with the
expectation of severe toxicity, in the hope of somewhat longer survival?
Would you agree to be treated under an experimental protocol, under

which you would be randomly assigned to receive either a new experimental drug or standard therapy in comparison to an inactive agent (placebo)?

Every day, many people and their families must face this most difficult of all decisions. Do you have the necessary knowledge, or information, on which to base such a decision? Does your physician, for that matter? In the constant search for improved treatment, many of the chemotherapy regimens recommended to patients are necessarily experimental in character, that is, their outcome is not yet known. It is hoped that their results will be superior to those of existing treatments. The outcome actually may be poorer. Yet the rules governing experimental studies on human subjects require that the patient give informed consent to the proposed treatment.

The rules have their origin in the trials of German war criminals at Nuremberg in 1945–1946. Among the criminals were Nazi doctors who had carried out cruel, even hideous, experiments on captives in the concentration camps. Certainly, the medical profession had been perverted in a state such as Nazi Germany. So had the judges, lawyers, professors, and most of society for that matter, so that no one can say it could not happen elsewhere. The doctors' trials have been recounted by William L. Shirer,[1] and are available in published transcripts of the proceedings.[2] The principle has derived from these trials that voluntary consent of the subject is absolutely essential in human experimentation, defined for a peacetime world by the Declaration of Helsinki: "The potential subject must be adequately informed of the aims, anticipated benefits, and potential hazards of the study, and of the discomfort or risk it may entail."[3] Further: "Concern for the interests of the subject must always prevail over the interests of science and of society." In the United States today, every hospital at which clinical studies are conducted must establish and maintain its Institutional Review Board For Protection of Human Subjects, composed not only of physicians but of representatives from the clergy, the legal profession, and the public. No study may be conducted on patients without prior formal consideration and approval by the review board. Practically speaking, each member of the board holds power of veto over any of the projects submitted to it.

Are the patients, and potential research subjects, ever in a position to understand what a physician is saying, able to give informed consent? Their level of understanding cannot be the same as that of the investigator, and they have little choice but to accept what the investigator tells them about the disease. There may be subtle pressures applied to patients to agree. Without firsthand knowledge of medicine, it is unlikely that they can make the kind of decision that the law would regard as informed.

A very few studies have been done entirely upon volunteer physicians, as was the smoking study conducted by the British Medical Association among its members and the recent United States study of aspirin in the prevention of heart attacks.[4] Physicians are a small segment of society, so that clinical research would slow to a crawl, or stop, if it had to depend on them alone. It is important to understand that patients who agree to take part in clinical trials are not giving up their rights to the best of medical care; on the contrary, they are likely to receive the closest attention from their physicians. Patients who participated in prospective, randomized trials of adjuvant treatment for non-small-cell carcinoma of the lung were found by one study to have better survival than did the patients who did not participate (P < 0.001). Favorable survival was noted in all groups of the trial patients, whether they had been randomly assigned to receive experimental therapy, or to be controls receiving either standard therapy or a placebo.[5] No explanation for this finding makes sense, unless it is that these patients received closer and more personal supportive attention from their doctors, because they were included in a study, than did those who had declined to participate.

Do patients ever suffer from their participation in a study? Such a possibility exists, but the mechanism of review is intended to minimize it, reduce it to as close to zero as possible. Yet chemotherapy for lung cancer seeks to prolong survival in an incurable stage of disease. It cannot possibly succeed if given at minimal dosage, at a level that could not harm or inconvenience the patient, but it may have more success if pushed to the point of actually endangering the patient by causing toxicity. Surgical treatment carries a distinct hazard, one which is accepted in exchange for a possibility of cure in properly selected cases. Chemotherapy trials suffer by comparison since treatment is not potentially curative, except in small-cell carcinoma, so that the possibility of fatal toxicity is more difficult to accept. In the early period of combined modality treatment for small-cell carcinoma, when a high proportion of complete remissions began to appear, many investigators saw promise of eventual cures. The question then became: Would more cures be achieved by treating patients to the absolute limits of their tolerance, disregarding risk, or by treating them within limits that they could easily stand? One regimen in particular, notable for its ferocity, caused the death of almost one-quarter of the treated patients from toxicity, or from direct complications of treatment.[6] In the end, the treatment had fewer long survivors than did other programs which had caused no fatalities.

Doubtful utility of chemotherapy at present for non-small-cell carcinoma of the lung was underscored by a recent study of physician attitudes toward treatment.[7] One hundred and eighteen physicians of the Ontario Cancer Research and Treatment Foundation were polled, of which seventy-nine responded. (The Foundation is largely responsible for cancer treatment, mainly nonsurgical treatment, throughout the province of Ontario.) Ninety-one percent of the responders spent at least 80 percent of their time treating cancer, primarily lung cancer patients. Fifty-one were graduates of United States or Canadian medical schools, twenty-five had been educated in Great Britain, and three in other countries. The majority practiced medical oncology or radiation therapy, with the remainder made up of a few thoracic surgeons and medical pulmonary-disease specialists. Four different scenarios were presented to the panel, each assuming that the physician had been found to have lung cancer. Details were specified of cell type, stage, and symptoms. Randomized protocols for cancer treatment appropriate to that tumor stage, which were already in existence in Canada or the United States, were given together with the question of whether the physician would agree to be entered in them, or would refuse. Acceptance of the protocols by these cancer specialists ranged from 11 percent to 64 percent of responders. Generally, the answers reflected complete acceptance of surgical resection as treatment for localized disease, but a considerable refusal to accept randomization to receive chemotherapy, even for widespread disease. Medical specialty of the responders had relatively little effect on their acceptance of individual protocols. Of the seventy-nine responding physicians, twenty-three were or had been habitual smokers; the smokers appeared to be more discriminating in their choices, suggesting that they already had considered these possibilities.

The authors noted that this panel of experts had rendered a devastating adverse verdict upon experimental cancer treatment as it is widely conducted, since they would not accept for themselves many of the chemotherapy protocols already in existence. Fundamentally, the verdict reflects disillusion with results of chemotherapy for non-small-cell lung cancer. Its conclusions have been echoed by other oncologists, one of whom wrote in an editorial, "Based on the existing literature, it is difficult not to concur with our colleagues."[8] The dilemma of the oncologist is whether treatment by chemotherapy should be advised at all for the patient with advanced non-small-cell carcinoma of the lung—at least until newer and more promising methods become available. But more promising methods will not be discovered, except through continued studies of experimental chemotherapy. What should patients, lay people, do when confronted with the question of treatment? First, they should ask for a full explanation of the difficulties, the possible adverse effects, of the proposed treatment, and also for an honest estimate of the chances of benefit. Another independent professional opinion often helps to put the decision into proper perspective. Several days or more may be necessary to think over the question and to discuss it with family and friends. Patients have the final word in all decisions about treatment. They should not ever feel that they are being pressured to agree. Ultimately, individual factors will control the decision, and no two people are likely to respond in exactly the same way. Patients may decide to refuse treatment, as is their right. In such a deadlock, the continuing support of a compassionate personal physician is of the greatest importance. One's own doctor is likely to have the resources and strength which the patient may need the most later on.

Some persons dislike and distrust doctors in general and will seek the help of charlatans instead. It is natural for patients and their families to clutch at straws when the medical profession can offer no possibility of cure. We must discuss this further in Chapter 18.

Sixteen

PRODUCT LIABILITY

Up in Smoke: A Jury Snuffs a Cigarette Suit
So attached to cigarettes was John Galbraith, 69, that
even while hospitalized with lung cancer, heart disease, and emphysema, he would slip off his oxygen
mask to sneak a smoke. Before death ended his 51–
year, three-pack-a-day habit in 1982, Galbraith had
filed a $1 million product-liability suit against R. J.
Reynolds. . . . But last week a jury . . . of eleven
nonsmokers and one smoker agreed with Reynolds's
attorney Thomas Workman that Galbraith "smoked
because he loved it. He knew the risks involved and
took them."

—*Time* magazine, January 6, 1986

Suppose that Mr. Galbraith's suit against R. J. Reynolds had been tried
before a jury of twelve habitual smokers, would the verdict have been
different? If the jury had been made up of twelve ex-smokers all of whom
had quit, what then? Or of twelve persons who had never smoked?
Presumably at least one juror from each category took part in the actual
verdict, although the account does not tell us specifically that any were
ex-smokers. Much is being said in the media about a new flood of
product-liability lawsuits which will threaten the tobacco companies
with ruin. Dr. Bill Hunter, for one, doubts that cigarette manufacturers
will ever be bankrupted by the predicted deluge. His estimate is that all
groups, smokers, ex-smokers, and nonsmokers, retain sufficient consciousness of individual responsibility that frequent unanimous jury verdicts for the plaintiffs will be unlikely.

Before June 1988, no cigarette manufacturer had been held financially responsible to a plaintiff for product liability, that is, for the plaintiff's death or illness from disease caused by smoking. Since the verdict in *Galbraith* v. *R. J. Reynolds*, numerous other actions continue to be brought against tobacco companies, most of them reported in detail by the press. In 1986, a young widow in upstate New York filed suit against Philip Morris Inc. and Lorillard Inc. for $20 million in the death of her husband, a prominent attorney and former city councilman. The suit claimed that the companies' advertising "enticed" him to continue smoking until he died of lung cancer at the age of forty-six. The suit, however, was dropped in 1987.

In January 1988 a jury in Lexington, Mississippi failed by a vote of 7 to 5 to reach a verdict in the case of *Horton* v. *American Tobacco Company*, the makers of Pall Mall cigarettes. Suit had been brought by Nathan H. Horton, and continued by his widow Ella Mae Horton after his death from lung cancer in January 1987, at the age of fifty. Mr. Horton had smoked two packs of cigarettes per day for most of his life. The suit asked damages of $17 million. This case had appeared to be unusually favorable for the plaintiff; the action had received strong support from the new Tobacco Products Liability Project, formed in 1985 with the aim of breaking the historic invulnerability of the tobacco companies to liability judgments. The project's director, Professor Richard Daynard of Northeastern University Law School, had sought to bring together concerned lawyers, thoracic surgeons, and cancer specialists to attack the problem, and to establish a central information exchange upon which all participants could draw.[1] The liability project may have increasing influence upon the course of similar actions in the future.

On June 13, 1988, a jury in Newark, N.J., reached a verdict in the case of *Cipollone* v. *Liggett Group, Lorillard Inc. and Philip Morris Inc.*, the first judgment ordering payment to a plaintiff by defendant tobacco companies. This case in particular had been supported heavily by the Tobacco Products Liability Project. The plaintiff, Rose Cipollone, had begun smoking at age sixteen and had smoked one and a half to two packs a day for forty-two years.[2] It was said that from the early 1950s onward, her husband and children "repeatedly" tried to get her to quit, but that she ignored their pleas. In 1981 she was found to have lung cancer and underwent surgical removal of the right upper lobe. In 1982 local recurrence of the tumor was found, and the remainder of the right lung was removed. She continued to smoke for another year after this, but quit approximately a year before her death from lung cancer at age fifty-eight in 1984. In August 1983, she had filed suit for unspecified damages against three cigarette manufacturers, and following her death the suit was continued by her husband.

In 1984, after the filing of her suit, Mrs. Cipollone was quoted by the press as saying, "I was sure that if there was anything that dangerous, that the tobacco people wouldn't allow it, and the government wouldn't let them sell cigarettes." By this time a vested interest on her part may be discerned. Previously, she had testified in a deposition that she smoked because she enjoyed it, despite warnings from her family, the Surgeon General, and many published reports in the press.[3]

"Mrs. Cipollone made a decision you and I make every day of our lives: to do, or not to do, something that is risky," said Peter K. Bleakly to the court on June 2, 1988. (Bleakly was an attorney for Philip Morris Inc.) Trial court, obviously, functions on the adversarial system. "The doctors couldn't get her to stop. Her husband couldn't get her to stop. She wasn't going to take orders from anybody," said Donald Cohn (attorney for the Liggett Group).

A brief review of chronology is necessary here in order to clarify the verdict. Following the Surgeon General's Report in 1964, Congress passed a law in 1965 requiring all cigarette packs and advertisements to carry a warning label; the law went into effect on January 1, 1966. Subsequent legal decisions have maintained that because of the warnings, the tobacco companies are no longer liable for injuries suffered after that date. Only the Liggett Group, makers of the now defunct Chesterfield brand, was held liable for any injury to Mrs. Cipollone since she had smoked Chesterfields before 1966. Lorillard and Philip Morris were exempted from liability. After hearing repeated testimony that Mrs. Cipollone had been aware of the dangers of smoking, the jury found her 80 percent responsible for her illness, and Lorillard 20 percent responsible. Since New Jersey law requires that the defendant be at least 50 percent responsible in product-liability suits, the jury made no award to Rose Cipollone's estate. An award of $400,000 was made to her husband, called by the defense "an expression of sympathy by the jury." All the defendant tobacco companies were found not guilty of additional charges of conspiracy and fraudulent misrepresentation. Both sides in the trial claimed the verdict as a victory, and appeals were filed promptly on behalf of the defendant companies. But this was the first time, among approximately 300 lawsuits filed against them since 1954, that the tobacco companies had been ordered to pay a judgment.

Most observers believe that the jury pussyfooted around the real issue: Who was responsible? The columnist James J. Kilpatrick ridiculed the idea of "80 percent responsibility," calling the plaintiff's case "The Devil Made Me Do It Syndrome": "Why, then, didn't Rose Cipollone quit? Why don't all smokers quit? The answer is that she simply didn't want to quit, not in her heart of hearts, not really and truly. But to accept that hard truth isn't easy."[4]

Rose Cipollone's lawyer, Marc Z. Edell, heavily supported by the Tobacco Products Liability Project, had claimed helpless addiction as the reason for her inability to give up smoking. The problem of addiction to cigarettes is central to the issue. From the legal standpoint: Should addiction free a person from the legal consequences of his or her acts, as insanity is held to do? To date, no M 'Naghten Rule grants the addicted person absolution from the consequences.

The painful crux of the matter is that a confirmed smoker loves his cigarettes, cannot stand to be without them. But it is possible to quit, cold turkey and of one's own volition. Then exactly where does the legal liability stand for illness and death caused by tobacco use? Is it with the tobacco companies? Are their profits not blood money, seeing that the product has a cumulative lethal effect? Certainly they are. Then why should the companies not be taxed out of existence? The United States government, like others, unfortunately has a financial stake in the continued use of cigarettes. Why should the companies not be bankrupted by liability suits? Unfortunately, it seems impossible that consumption of cigarettes would disappear in the United States, any more than the consumption of liquor disappeared during Prohibition. Distribution and sale of cigarettes surely would fall into the hands of the criminal underground, with profits so great that courts and police departments could be corrupted as they were during the 1920s. Could the criminal underground be sued successfully, for "wrongful death" of the smokers, as tobacco companies are now? Most observers, Bill Hunter among them, regretfully conclude that there can be no easy answer for the massive problem of lung cancer. Many of them hope that public education can be made more effective, by emphasizing individual responsibility for prevention. We have seen that treatment has limited effectiveness, and only prevention can help. Certainly the problem is too important to be left to the doctors, or even to the lawyers.[5]

Will there be more, larger, Cipollone-type verdicts? The tobacco industry can probably survive them. Although per capita cigarette con-

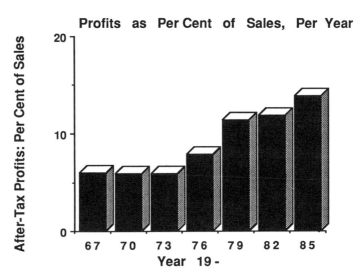

*Figure 16.1. Yearly after-tax profits of U. S. cigarette manufacturers, as percent of sales. (*Source: *U. S. Department of Agriculture.)*

sumption in the United States is declining, profits are rising because of price increases and booming sales in Third World countries (fig. 16.1). The industry's revenues in 1987 totaled $32 billion, with predicted earnings of $6.4 billion in 1988 (1986 earnings were $5.2 billion.) It is estimated that the United States tobacco companies could lose fifteen thousand verdicts a year like Cipollone's and pay the entire $6 billion in damages simply by raising the price of cigarettes twenty-five cents per pack, even allowing for a 10 percent drop in sales in the United States because of the higher price. The average cost of a pack in the United States in 1988 was $1.24, compared to sixty-six cents in 1981.

Will education of the public be effective enough, to begin to control lung cancer by prevention? Within the past decade, a considerable change in lifestyle has become visible in the United States, and there is much diminished tolerance of smoking in public places. Presumably the greatest difficulty will be to prevent acquisition of the habit by young people, teenagers in particular. As long as young people continue to see smoking as a metaphor for maturity, sophistication, sexual experience, worldly knowledge, and the like, there will be early fixation of the habit on large numbers of persons who later will be unwilling to give it up. The legal issue for the future is whether these persons must later be accountable for their own actions, or whether liability rests with the companies that sold them cigarettes.

Seventeen

ADDICTION

If you do not wish to take the drug again, you tell
yourself, you need not do so. As an intelligent person
you are superior to the stuff. Then there is no logical
reason why you should not enjoy yourself again, is
there? Of course there isn't! And so you do. But this
time it is a little disappointing. Your half a gramme
was not quite enough. Disappointment must be dealt
with. You must wander in Paradise just once more
before you decide not to take the stuff again. A trifle
more; nearly a gramme perhaps. Paradise again and
still you don't feel any the worse for it. So why not
continue? The moment you detect any bad effects,
you *will* stop. Only fools become addicts.

—Eric Ambler, *A Coffin for Dimitrios* (1939)

Compulsive use of tobacco has been observed in practically every culture
to which tobacco has been introduced. All tobacco products contain
substantial amounts of nicotine and other alkaloids; they are present in
living or dried tobacco leaf, "smokeless" preparations such as snuff and
chewing tobacco, and all smoking varieties. The term *alkaloids* in the
present context signifies a group of compounds of plant origin, mildly
basic in pure form, with powerful physiologic effects in the body. Nicotine
is the primary addicting substance in tobacco; chemically it is a tertiary
amine, an organic compound derived in structure from the ammonia
molecule (NH_3), but with all three hydrogen atoms replaced by alkyl
groups. The molecule's structure includes two joined rings, of different
configurations. Nicotine is readily absorbed into the bloodstream from
tobacco smoke in the lungs, or from smokeless tobacco in the mouth or

nose. It may be absorbed through the skin; agricultural workers occasionally are subject to nicotine toxicity from contact with moist tobacco leaves.[1] Nicotine entering the blood is rapidly distributed to the brain, where it binds to chemical receptors located throughout the nervous sytem. It induces relaxation in skeletal muscle and has effects on nearly all the endocrine or internal-secreting glands. In regular tobacco users, nicotine levels accumulate in the body during the day and persist at declining levels overnight; as a result, daily users maintain some degree of exposure to the drug practically around the clock. Nicotine use during at least the previous twenty-four hours can be verified by analyzing urine for the presence of the primary metabolic product, cotinine.

Benefits claimed for the smoking habit include pleasurable relaxation, euphoria, relief of tension especially at times of stress, improvement in attention time and ability to concentrate. To what extent these represent only alleviation of withdrawal symptoms—fatigue, anxiety, irritability, sleeplessness, and the like, is at least partly a question of definitions.[2] Smokers also develop a habitual pattern of motor activity which is familiar and reassuring, a constantly present support. Smoking in public offers many people a relief from worries and uncertainty, something to do, a usually acceptable method of reducing tension precipitated by social pressures or feelings of inadequacy.[3]

Smokers consistently maintain a relatively constant nicotine intake from day to day; they will increase consumption of "low-yield" cigarettes to maintain the accustomed nicotine intake. Volunteer smokers can differentiate between cigarettes that vary in their delivery of nicotine and can clearly differentiate nicotine from a placebo. A degree of chronic tolerance to the drug develops in all regular users; that is, the user gradually requires larger amounts of intake in order to maintain the desired effects.[4] Two other effects are more indicative of subjects' true capacity for addiction. First is the mechanism called "positive reinforcement." Drugs can serve as stimuli which strengthen behavior leading to further presentation of the drug. Animals, for example, quickly learn to manipulate levers that deliver additional doses of narcotic drugs to them. The strongest such stimuli in the human smoker are likely to be pleasure and relief from withdrawal symptoms.

"Withdrawal Reactions"—the second effect—become clear signs of physical dependence. Termination of smoking, for example, is accompanied by depressive changes in mood, behavior, and physical functioning. All these changes are opposite to those produced by smoking. An important point is that physiologic withdrawal effects can be reversed by nicotine administration in other ways, such as by nicotine chewing gum. Nicotine gum, paradoxically, sometimes maintains physical dependence in ex-smokers, instead of breaking it.

Positive reinforcement and withdrawal reactions: do these constitute a definition of drug dependence? The word *dependence* has largely replaced the word *addiction* in medical terminology.[5] A consensus definition would be that the psychoactive drug has come to control behavior to an extent that is detrimental to the individual or society. Involvement of a psychoactive drug is the critical feature that distinguishes drug addictions from other habitual behavior. The *Diagnostic and Statistical Manual,* third edition (DSM-III), of the American Psychiatric Association says, "The essential feature of the disorder is a cluster of cognitive, behavioral, and physiological symptoms that indicate that the person has impaired control of psychoactive substance use and continues use of the substance despite adverse consequences."[6] Ten classes of psychoactive substances are designated: the amphetamine group of compounds (including "speed," "bennies," and "dexies"); cannabis, or marijuana; cocaine; hallucinogens such as peyote; inhalants such as aromatic glues and solvents; nicotine; opium-derived narcotics such as morphine and heroin; the class of PCP-like compounds ("angel dust" and its derivatives); and the class of sleeping pills, sedatives, and tranquilizers. Tobacco use concurrent with other drug dependencies is so prevalent that it is not generally considered to be of diagnostic significance, or considered as a basis for diagnosis of multiple-drug dependency.

TREATMENT PROGRAMS

Because cigarette smoking, like other forms of drug dependence, involves both pharmacological and behavioral factors, many believe that treatment strategies should include pharmacologic agents, behavioral strategies, or combinations of the two. The fact remains that most ex-smokers had quit the habit spontaneously and alone.[7] A 1985 national survey estimated the number of former smokers in the United States at approximately 41 million. Ninety percent of the former smokers surveyed reported that they had quit without formal treatment programs or smoking-cessation devices.[8] A comparison of thirty-nine reported trials of smoking cessation concluded that treatment programs were most effective if they employed more than one modality for motivating behavioral change, involved both physicians and nonphysicians in an individualized face-to-face effort, and reinforced the motivational message on multiple occasions over the longest possible time period.[9] It is dismaying to note that most reports of smoking-cessation programs report their results after a period of only six months. After one year, the proportion of persons continuing to abstain is considerably lower; reported proportions range from 5 or 6 percent to a few as high as 17 to 20 percent. The relapse rate after formal cessation programs remains high. Is spontaneous resolution to quit any better? No really accurate comparative figures can be developed, but the great majority of those people who have been able to quit spontaneously had previously made one or more unsuccessful efforts.[10] From whatever standpoint, the highly dependent smoker has a relatively intractable problem.

A recent study of 380 smokers participating in a smoking relapse prevention trial divided the subjects into those with "heavy" usage (twenty-five or more cigarettes per day) or "light" usage (fifteen or fewer cigarettes per day). "Heavy" smokers reported greater difficulty quitting, were more troubled by withdrawal symptoms, experienced stronger urgings and cravings, and had significantly higher scores on responses to a questionnaire designed to assess tobacco dependence. Not surprisingly, the study concluded that heavy smokers are more dependent on cigarettes, thus presumably more severely addicted.[11]

A question remains about the 35 million or so smokers in the United States who have broken the habit spontaneously and by their own resolve. Many of them, as Bill Hunter can vouch for himself, maintained long-term consumption of more than twenty-five cigarettes per day and would have been classed in the study discussed as heavy, dependent smokers. Is nicotine addiction comparable to heroin or cocaine addiction, as is often claimed? The two forms of dependence are different in many ways, but a survey of multiple-drug users suggested that they regard tobacco addiction as relatively difficult to break.[12] On the other hand, no evidence exists that anything like 35 to 40 million cocaine or heroin addicts have been able to break the habit, by any method, and abstain thereafter.

What should heavy smokers do, who need badly to break the habit, and who in all likelihood have already tried a couple of times but unsuccessfully? The available figures indicate strongly that their best chance will be to do it by themselves. Does that mean they will need tremendous willpower? At least one thoughtful observer has pointed out that what they really need is motivation, not by any means the same thing as simple willpower.[13] Why is that so different? "Motivation" in this context means that the smoker must have a good and compelling reason for wanting to quit. Simply wanting to quit is not enough; the great majority of heavy smokers tell the interviewer that yes, of course they want to quit, but have not been able to. Smokers have been motivated to quit by the onset of a sudden smoking-related illness, such as a myocardial infarction or heart attack; by having seen a friend or associate struck down by lung cancer; by an awareness of increasing smoker's cough or a diminished breathing capacity on their own part; by realization of how much a spouse or children depend upon them; sometimes by disgust with what has begun to appear a filthy habit, or with their own dependence upon it. Sometimes a person's own physician has given an ultimatum: quit smoking, or find another doctor. In the bluntest of terms, any sudden and cogent reminder of one's own mortality, and of its relation to smoking, seems to be the most effective stimulus. Tragically, the reminder of mortality may come too late. The important point is that the motive can come only from the smoker. It cannot be added temporarily, like a crutch; and unless the smoker can find an adequate motive for quitting, almost any externally applied program is likely to fail.[14]

Fearing that one lacks sufficient motivation to make the drastic, wrenching turnabout alone, what should a person do who wishes to quit? Discussion with one's own physician is a useful first step. The physician may choose to reinforce his or her advice to the patient personally, on repeated occasions; or the physician may have the patient enroll in voluntary abstinence programs. Group support, and public commitments to abstain, probably are of variable importance, depending on the individual's personality traits. The value of nicotine gum as a substitute during the withdrawal period remains uncertain, although many physicians would probably advise it. Most importantly, repeated attempts to quit may eventually lead to success, as many ex-smokers attest, and perseverance may well be of value.

Eighteen

UNORTHODOX OR "ALTERNATIVE" TREATMENT

It is necessary to the happiness of man that he be mentally faithful to himself. Infidelity does not consist in believing, or in disbelieving; it consists in professing to believe what one does not believe.

—Thomas Paine, *The Age of Reason* (1797)

It ain't what a man don't know that makes him a fool, but what he does know that ain't so.

—Josh Billings (Henry Wheeler Shaw)
(1818–1885)

WHAT DO I HAVE TO LOSE?

Every time a doctor must tell a patient or family that there can be no real chance of curing a particular case of cancer, many are likely to misinterpret the words and hear instead the message, "Nothing can be done." Few doctors say that, if any, because in the situation of last resort there often are possibilities of treatment for palliation; or, if nothing else, of personal support and continuing concern from the physician so that the patient need not feel abandoned. But whether a patient hears these words, or only imagines having heard them, his or her mind often runs to well-remembered stories of a neighbor's uncle or cousin who went instead to Mexico or to the Bahamas and received a miraculous cure, which is forbidden in the United States because the "medical monopoly" is opposed to it. The patient comes to the instant conclusion, "What do I have to lose?" and the stage is set for the resort to quackery.

Many people dislike and distrust physicians for a variety of reasons. Those who are imbued with the philosophy of "natural healing," with the concept that "you are what you eat," or of "mind over body," or of the "right to choose" one's own treatment, may be unwilling to accept medical treatment even during the stage when the cancer might be treatable with hope of a cure. They have a ready ear for pejorative descriptions of surgery as "butchery" or "hacking"; of radiation therapy as "burning out your insides"; or of chemotherapy as "poisoning your system." They will listen to the voices of popular wisdom which say that you have to go outside the country in order to get "natural" or effective treatment for cancer. What do they have to lose, indeed? First, the possibility of cure in at least a few cases, or of prolongation of life in at least some more. Those who dislike physicians, believing them to be greedy and mercenary, getting rich at the expense of the sick patient, have seen nothing until they have been to the clinics of alternative treatment.

It is their own choice and right to do so. By all means; patients have the right to refuse any treatment advised to them by physicians. Then why should we worry if some patients choose an unorthodox or unproved method of treatment? Let us not worry. Our intent is to look objectively at the problem of lung cancer, difficult and adverse though it may be. One concern should be against the raising of unreasonable hopes in the patient and the family, which are bound to be dashed; another, against the extraction of their resources, without provision in return of scientifically grounded treatment or investigation, which must be so represented to them at the time.

Scientific inquiry is based upon skepticism of easy answers, upon the controlled experiment, and open publication of findings in journals after review by the investigator's peers. Although scientific inquiry has not yet found the "cure for cancer" desired by the media as being easy to take, invariably effective, and with no aftereffects, the truth remains now as ever that "no free lunch" is available. Biologic science still seeks for basic understanding of the life processes; as this is gained, medicine should begin to approach the possibility of reliable cure without serious aftereffects, a result which can be attained only occasionally and unpredictably at present. But how can we recognize fraudulence and humbug? If the patient or family are doubtful or fearful of medical advice given them regarding treatment, how can they tell whether the alternative practitioner's method is based upon secure knowledge and record, or upon moonshine and folktales? I offer several criteria for deciding; if these are clearly evident, distrust the practitioner:

1. Patients come to the practitioner not as a result of referral from their own or any other physician, but as the result of word-of-mouth recommendations through the natural-healing subculture. Referral of the patient to a regional cancer center, on the other hand, will have been made by the physician on the grounds of published results of treatment of that type of disease.

2. Publicity for the alternative treatment has been spread through testimonials, published in "health" magazines or in pamphlets and flyers, rather than through publication in peer-reviewed medical journals. "What is wrong with that?" the critic will ask. "Don't you think those people are telling the truth in their testimonials? What reason would they have to lie about it?" All are questions that should answer themselves upon objective consideration, but seem to damn conventional treatment in the emotion-laden milieu in which they are asked.

   The alternative practitioner or clinic rarely if ever wishes to document the disease process with certainty, as by biopsy in the case of cancer. How many of the glowing testimonials came from people who actually did have cancer, or were only afraid they might? Because, let us say, they had been long-time heavy smokers? No one can ever know. The patients giving the testimonials: were they followed for five years, or for the otherwise appropriate periods, before having been pronounced cured? I have mentioned the surgeon-patient who appreciated the mental exercises of imagery and mastery over his cancer, but who succumbed to it all the same. Readers will recall another celebrity, Steve McQueen (1930–1980), who went to Mexico for much-publicized treatment and died there in 1980. The questions could go on and on. Follow-up and documentation are the keys to objective analysis of cancer treatment.

3. There is a very large payment required from the patient up front, not without frequent additional payments along the way.

4. The practitioner insists that his treatment (formula; ingredients; whatever) must be kept a secret, and he may not divulge them by open publication because they would be pirated by his opponents. This simply is not the way that science works. Only in, say, a

Manhattan Project to develop an atom bomb must scientific findings be kept secret for reasons of compelling national security. In
biological or medical science, secrecy has no place.

5. Most importantly, the practitioner makes sure all patients understand that "organized medicine (or the medical establishment) is
against me because the success of my treatment will diminish their
profits. That's why 'they' won't let me give this treatment in the
United States, and you have to come to (offshore, wherever) to get
it." This allegation in particular finds ready acceptance and belief
among members of the alternative-treatment subculture. Is it true?
Let's not try to answer yes or no. The Socratic method of inquiry
would be to examine the consequences which would follow if the
hypothesis were true.

Dr. Bill Hunter has seen two professors of surgery in his department
die of lung cancer since he first became a faculty member, as well as
several practicing physicians whom he had seen in consultation. He has
seen several physicians' wives die, either of lung cancer itself or of metastases to the lungs from cancer elsewhere. Are physicians, or their families, immune to death from cancer? Unless the answer is yes, how could
the profession possibly wish to suppress new treatments that offer promise for improved survival? Outside Bill's own medical school, a number of
world-renowned professors and chairmen of departments of surgery
have died of lung cancer. Several of them are among the authors cited in
the bibliography. Would these men have been part of the "medical establishment" and therefore intent on suppressing new or alternative treatments? The reader should decide the truth of the alternative-treatment
practitioner's charge on the basis of these consequences.

SOME UNPROVED TREATMENTS

It would not be possible to list all the nostrums that have been peddled to
the public as cures for cancer, but anyone of approximately Bill Hunter's
age will remember several whose proprietors sought and received
strident national publicity. There was the Hoxsey Clinic of Dallas, Texas,
and the Hoxsey Method of Cancer Treatment.[1] Harry Hoxsey was not a
physician (his formal education terminated during the eighth grade), but
had peddled his elixirs throughout the Midwest beginning in the 1920s.
His clinic in Dallas opened in 1936. Eventually a permanent injunction

was obtained by the Food and Drug Administration in September 1960, banning sale of the Hoxsey "medications" by his clinic and its successor, but testimonials of patients claiming to have been cured of cancer continued to appear for some years in health magazines. The magazines also continued to publish formulas for the Hoxsey "medications," together with names and addresses of herbalists from whom the ingredients could be obtained.

The cancer treatment of Dr. Max Gerson of New York was described as a method of: (1) "detoxification of the whole body," by daily administration of coffee enemas, so as to produce at least one copious bowel movement per day; (2) providing "essential components of the potassium group"; and (3) "adding oxidizing enzymes continuously, as long as they are not being built in the body," in the form of a diet composed principally of green-leaf juices and fresh calves' liver juice. Gerson and later promoters have learned to describe their arcana in terms that sound impressively scientific to the public. Gerson acquired a devoted group of followers who saw the millennium arriving, but who gradually dispersed after his death in 1959 and after objective examinations of his claims.[2]

Two classics in cancer quackery are the sagas of Krebiozen and Laetrile. The former allegedly was brought to this country from Argentina by a Yugoslav physician, Dr. Stevan Durovic, and his brother Marko, described as a lawyer and industrialist. Its nature and composition remained a jealously guarded secret. Widely promoted and sold to both patients and physicians, it acquired an impressive list of partisans including Dr. Andrew C. Ivy, a professor emeritus of physiology and vice-president of the University of Illinois, and Senator Paul Douglas.[3] The Food and Drug Administration (FDA), strengthened in its regulatory powers after the thalidomide episode, eventually required Durovic to file an acceptable plan for distribution of Krebiozen as an investigational drug. Upon his refusal, the preparation was barred from interstate distribution but continued to be sold freely in Illinois. Empowered also to analyze the material, the FDA found samples labeled as pure Krebiozen to contain only a common body chemical, creatine monohydrate, and mineral oil. Later samples contained mineral oil only. Subsequently Dr. Stevan Durovic fled the United States under indictment for income-tax evasion in the amount of $904,907 for the years 1960–1962 alone, and did not return. His brother Marko was served with a tax lien of more than half a million dollars for taxes which the Internal Revenue Service contended were not paid for the period 1954–1958. It appears that Dr.

Ivy also profited handsomely from his association with the Durovics,[4] although he was not indicted.

Laetrile, a phenomenon of the dominance of publicity over rational judgment, is unmatched in all this recital. Said to have been developed by a father and son, Ernest T. Krebs Senior and Junior, it was claimed to derive from the Unitarian or Trophoblastic Thesis of Cancer propounded by a John Beard of Edinburgh in 1902. (The words in the thesis's name are utterly without meaning in the context.) Krebs Senior, a doctor of medicine born in 1877, had extracted from apricot pits the cyanide-containing compound amygdalin as the essential ingredient. Later, this was named by his son, said to have been a "biochemist" but without a degree, "Vitamin B-17." A convoluted set of postulates was developed to the effect that the cyanide within the agent would be released only within cancer cells, killing them immediately.

The public's response to this hypothetical philosopher's stone was incredible, completely eclipsing any other unorthodox therapy ever used for any disease in our time.[5] Support and pressure groups sprang up; one, called the International Association of Cancer Victims and Friends (IACVF), was founded in 1963 by Cecile Hoffman, a cancer patient who believed that her life had been saved by the use of Laetrile. Mrs. Hoffman died later of metastatic cancer. Another was the Committee for Freedom of Choice in Cancer Therapy, Inc. (CFCCT), founded in California in 1962. The IACVF has sponsored a book, *World Without Cancer* and an hour-long documentary filmstrip by the same name, distributed by the CFCCT.[6] Numerous other books appeared, giving voice to a vehement, emotional partisanship. Laetrile was legalized by twenty-seven of the fifty states and also was sold nationwide in spite of the FDA restrictions, under a federal court order which had been reviewed by the Supreme Court but not reversed. A Harris poll found that the American public favored legalization on a national basis by an astounding margin of 30 percent.[7]

Lost in the furor has been the skeptic's question of whether it works. The National Cancer Institute (NCI) being a governmental agency, undertook first to review case histories submitted by Laetrile's backers but could find no evidence of benefit.[8] Subsequently, in order to lay the matter to rest, the NCI sponsored a clinical trial at several university medical centers, headed by the director of medical oncology at the Mayo Clinic. Conducted according to methods and dosages requested by Laetrile's partisans, and reported in complete and painstaking detail,[9] the trial found no evidence of benefit whatever. Even such a "trial" as this, brought about by public clamor and pressure from the public's representatives in Congress, was contrary to the scientific method. The National Cancer Institute's intramural rules require that preliminary testing of a new drug must show evidence of activity against cancer in animal systems before it is given a trial in patients, and no such data existed. Would the reader desire, as a cancer patient, to have been entered into the Laetrile trial because a political clamor had been raised that "the government should test it"?

More contemporaneous is the story of "Immuno-Augmentative Therapy" (IAT).[10] Lawrence Burton, not a physician but a Ph.D. in zoology, during the 1950s and 60s had studied proteins from leukemic mice which he reported had antitumor properties, and obtained four United States patents for methods by which different blood fractions were prepared. By adjusting the levels of these four fractions, he claimed to enable a patient's immune system to combat successfully any type of cancer. In 1974 he submitted to the Food and Drug Administration an application for testing of the blood fractions as investigational new drugs; but requests from the FDA for supporting data and information went unanswered, and the file was closed in 1976. Not being a physician, he could not be licensed to practice medicine, hence could not conduct clinical testing himself. In 1977 he moved to Freeport in the Bahama Islands and opened the Immunology Researching Center, where patients could come to receive his treatment, and it remains open.

New patients spend several weeks and an initial payment of $10,000 (U.S.) for their first treatment cycle at the clinic in Freeport. "Tests" are done, and each day filled syringes are delivered to the patients, who administer the material to themselves by subcutaneous or intramuscular injection. Later the patient is sent home with additional vials of the protein fractions and a schedule for self-administration. Patients are expected to return for periodic three- to five-day visits for reevaluation and additional treatments, with further payments each time.

In 1982 two state legislatures legalized the therapy, but one, Florida's, repealed the measure two years later. By 1983 patients with acquired immunodeficiency syndrome (AIDS) also were receiving IAT at the Burton clinic. In 1984 the Centers for Disease Control reported finding sixteen IAT patients with large, often multiple, abscesses at injection sites, caused by several strains of infecting organisms. Testing of the IAT materials by the National Cancer Institute found that all samples contained live bacteria, and, of those checked, all contained evidence of contamination by the hepatitis B virus. Additional testing by the state of Washington, of injectable materials given to patients at the Freeport clinic, found eight of eighteen samples contaminated by the human immunodeficiency virus, the cause of AIDS. No data have been released by Burton or his associates on the results of their treatment. Of a panel of expert consultants convened by the American Medical Association to review what is known of the Burton treatment, none believed its safety to be established, and 73 percent believed its safety to be unacceptable. None believed its effectiveness to be established, 22 percent listed its effectiveness currently as "investigational," and 59 percent rated it "unacceptable."[11]

THE RIGHT TO CHOOSE

Patients with early and potentially curable cancer—do they have the right to choose their own treatment if they distrust the advice they have been given? Of course, and they can refuse any or all treatment if they wish. Patients with advanced and incurable cancer—do they have the same right? Again, of course they do. This is the intensely emotional point upon which partisans of new or unorthodox therapies demand legalization of those treatments within the United States. Does the United States government, specifically the FDA, have the right to forbid use of that drug or treatment within the country? Now the question becomes more sticky.

Without the FDA, thousands of babies would have been born in the United States with deformed, flipper-like, or absent limbs. It did not happen because a conscientious FDA examiner refused to be hurried into approving thalidomide for marketing in the United States; in Europe, several thousand deformed babies were born. Do we expect our government to give us protection against unforeseen dangers, so far as that is possible? Without a doubt. Do we expect it to protect us against fraud?

"It's my life that is at stake, and my money that I will be paying. The doctors say nothing more can be done. Who has the right to tell me I can't get this treatment?" Do we still expect protection against fraud, or must we accept it as inevitable? And who is to say that it's fraud? Must we allow unscrupulous promoters to amass great wealth through the promotion of obvious fraud? Finally, do we need to be protected against ourselves?

Crusades to legalize any treatment by charlatans, at their own price, will in the end hurt the cancer patient most of all. At the very least, governmental regulation entails objective review of pertinent data on effectiveness as well as safety, and possible interdiction of those treatments unable to meet the review. We can't settle for less.

Nineteen

ECONOMICS, GOVERNMENT, AND THE MEDIA

We the People of the United States, in Order to form a more perfect Union, establish Justice, insure domestic Tranquility, provide for the common Defence, *promote the general Welfare,* and secure the Blessings of Liberty to ourselves and our Posterity, do ordain and establish this Constitution for the United States of America.

—Preamble to the Constitution of the United States (1787)

The Congress shall have Power to lay and collect Taxes, Duties, Imposts, and Excises, . . . To regulate Commerce . . . among the several States, and with the Indian Tribes.

—Constitution of the United States, Article I, Section 8

SMOKING AND THE PUBLIC WEAL

From first to last, tobacco has influenced our government. George Washington grew tobacco on his estate in Virginia. Ronald Reagan, while campaigning in North Carolina in 1980 for election to the presidency, promised his listeners what they wanted to hear: "My own Cabinet members will be far too busy with substantive matters to waste their time proselytizing against the dangers of cigarette smoking." Tobacco growing in the United States is geographically concentrated, east of the Mississippi River and south of the Mason-Dixon line; the six top-ranked states, all clustered in this area, produce three-quarters of the United States crop. Since Reconstruction, states of the Old South have been perceived to hold steadfast loyalty to their senators and congressmen in Washington, returning them in election after election. As a result, Southern senators in particular have tended to outlast their colleagues in seniority, and consequently to hold chairmanships of influential committees. Back in the home states, the income that a farmer can derive per acre from growing tobacco is more than ten times greater than he can obtain from growing corn or soybeans. A system of mandatory allotments of the acreage devoted to growing tobacco has stabilized the annual crop, and helps to maintain prices for the product.[1] Holders of allotments are assured of their market and income, an arrangement destructive of competition. Entirely apart from the influence of cigarette manufacturing companies, then, tobacco farming has wielded formidable political influence on the national scene. At issue for more than two decades has been the question of whether the United States should continue price supports to the farmers for growing a lethal product. The United States continues to do so, and not solely because of regional influence on the national government. There are other constraining reasons, almost never spoken of, which we must consider.

We already have reviewed the chronology of such restrictions as the United States government has placed on cigarette manufacturers. The Surgeon General's Report on Smoking and Health was released in 1964. Effective on January 1, 1966, Congress required labels on cigarette packages and in all advertisements, warning that cigarette smoking is hazardous to health. Effective January 1, 1971, cigarette advertising was banned from radio and television. In 1985, more strongly worded warnings were required, a list of four to be rotated every three months.

The total costs to the country of cigarette smoking, in terms of lost earnings, absenteeism, disability, forced retirement, and the like, are not borne primarily by the federal government. A survey in 1985 by the congressional Office of Technology Assessment concluded that the government of the United States pays approximately 4.2 billion dollars annually in smoking-related medical costs through Medicare, Medicaid, the Veterans' Administration hospital system, and the National Institutes of Health. This is the approximate direct bill, as the Congress sees it. There is the cost of price supports to the farmers, but it is minuscule by comparison.

Against this expenditure should be set, first, the receipt of federal and state cigarette taxes, estimated some years ago at $6 billion a year.[2] Since then, federal and many state taxes on cigarettes have been doubled, and more recent estimates had set receipts at approximately $12 billion per year. In early 1989, further increases were being actively discussed, as the Bush administration began to search for new sources of revenue that could be dismissed lightly as "sin taxes," or better yet as no taxes at all. Because of high and increasing sales to Third World countries, the federal government receives approximately $2.5 billion annually in export revenues.[3] But the greatest single benefit from a policy of laissez-faire is one that nobody likes to talk about.

In plain language, each current smoker in the United States will save the government a total of approximately $35,000 in Social Security payments, simply because the smokers will on the average die sooner than the nonsmokers.[4] The loss of life span represents a saving to the government of at least $10 billion per year for the next fifty years or so. Most of the premature deaths will occur after retirement and may not be due to cancer so much as to arteriosclerosis, heart disease, and chronic lung disease, the incidences of which are all increased by smoking. But many will still be due to lung cancer. In these days when the federal government runs at huge annual deficits, and talk of raising personal taxes amounts to political suicide in either the executive or the legislative branch, the Treasury Department holds this long range advantage into the future. It is unlikely that we will see cigarettes banned or taxed out of existence. And ours is not the only government embarrassed by the same problem: "The government in Britain could act by increasing the tax on tobacco, as did James I, (but).. the Treasury has decided that it is cost-effective to allow people to smoke themselves to death, rather than to look after them in their old age."[5]

CIGARETTE ADVERTISING

Should our government ban cigarette advertising entirely? Possibly—this move might have the advantage of cutting off from public exposure the image of glamor and sophistication with which the cigarette companies have so long invested their product. More than anything else, it might reduce the numbers of young people who are seduced into the habit in early life. Cigarette advertising was recently banned by the government of Canada (June 28, 1988), the prohibition to take effect at the beginning of 1989 for newspapers and magazines, in 1991 for billboard advertising, and in 1993 for retail store signs. While the ban surely will have to face legal challenges, on many grounds including that of freedom of speech, it has greatly encouraged anti-smoking advocates in the United States.

Figure 3.8 pointed out that annual per capita consumption of cigarettes in Canada was slightly higher even than that in the United States. Following passage of the ban, the Canadian minister of national health and welfare, Jake Epp, told the press that the law would end the tobacco industry's ability to portray smoking as socially acceptable or glamorous—at least within the country. "David finally slew Goliath," he said. Yet the movement for a ban had been gathering momentum for several years. Canada's oldest daily newspaper, the *Whig-Standard* of Kingston, Ontario, (circulation 37,000) announced on November 27, 1984, that after January 1 it would no longer accept cigarette advertising,[6] the first paper in the country to do so. Citing the precedent of the *Whig-Standard,* the *Recorder and Times* of Brockville, Ontario announced on April 12, 1985, that it too would not accept advertisements. This paper had found previously that its smoking employees lost more than twice as much time from work because of illness than did the nonsmokers, and in 1974 had banned smoking from its workplace. The publisher of Canada's national newspaper, *The Globe and Mail* of Toronto, at first declined to follow suit on grounds that to do so would infringe freedom of speech; but not long afterward joined in the ban on advertising together with *The Toronto Star,* Canada's largest-circulation newspaper.[7]

A few United States newspapers have never accepted tobacco advertising on grounds of religious belief, notably the *Deseret News* (Salt Lake City) and the *Christian Science Monitor* of Boston. In 1949, even before the report of Wynder and Graham, the publisher of the Sarasota, Florida, *Herald-Tribune and Journal* announced that his paper would no longer accept cigarette advertisements. He had become convinced of the relation between smoking and disease after his father had undergone a pneumonectomy for lung cancer. But in 1982, his policy was voided when the paper was purchased by the *New York Times;* the *Times* for many years has delighted to castigate the medical profession for avarice and greed, but itself continues to derive massive revenues from cigarette advertising.[8] A recent issue of the *Times* weekly magazine (July 10, 1988) featured a lead story by Peter Schmeisser entitled, "Pushing Cigarettes Overseas," complete with color layout on the cover. The subtitle read, "Even as the Surgeon General fights tobacco at home, U.S. trade officials press sales abroad." Inside were advertisements for the R. J. Reynolds Tobacco Company's (Now) and the American Tobacco Company's Carlton.

Time Magazine has done much the same. An issue some years ago (May 28, 1979) featured an analysis titled, "Medical Costs: Seeking the Cure." The cover picture showed a purported surgeon, capped and masked so that only his piercing eyes were exposed. The mask was imprinted with the design of a dollar bill, complete down to the likeness of George Washington. So far, so good; the picture was designed to prejudice the reader instantly. The back cover, part of the same sheet of paper and also in color, was a full-page advertisement for Camel cigarettes ("Introducing: The solution for 100's smokers.") Another issue featured a cover story, "Fighting Cocaine's Grip: Millions of Users; Billions of Dollars." Again, the back cover was a full-page cigarette advertisement ("Expect Taste . . . Nothing halfway about it. MERIT.") A cover story in *Newsweek*, "How Good Is Your Doctor?" depicted three grim-looking characters, again garbed as surgeons, with scalpels, forceps, and scissors in hand, glaring down upon the inferred patient. The back cover was a full-page advertisement in color for Pall Mall Gold 100's. All three of these periodicals have thanked cigarette companies in the pages of the *United States Tobacco Journal* and other trade organs for their continued heavy support through advertising.

The group of magazines aimed primarily for women are a specially illustrative case. Until about 1965, cigarette advertising hardly existed in them. But a tabulation of the pages of cigarette advertising in the *Ladies' Home Journal* found that during the year 1960, two pages of cigarette ads had appeared in 2,022 total pages, approximately 0.1 percent.[9] In 1970, pages of cigarette advertising had increased to 17 out of 1,856, about 0.9 percent; in 1975, to 111 out of 1,690 or 6.5 percent; and in 1980 to 180 of 2,044 or 8.8 percent. The pages devoted to cigarette advertising had increased almost a hundredfold. Over the same years, annual women's lung cancer death rates increased from six to twenty-two per 100,000, or by 367 percent. Yet the magazines continue to derive large incomes from cigarette advertising. A front-page article in *Advertising Age*, "Women Top Cig Target," (in 1981) quoted the president and chief executive officer of R. J. Reynolds describing the women's market as "probably the largest opportunity" for the company.[10] Another article in the same journal (in 1983) was "Marketers Clamor to Offer Lady A Cigarette."[11] Several new brands of cigarettes have appeared, intended specifically for marketing to women. "When Virginia Slims hit the market, at about the same time as feminism became an issue, American Womanhood was primed for a cigarette it could call its own."[12] "Good-oh!" was Bill Hunter's reaction on reading this. "Who says you can't have it all?"

Only a few magazines have refused to carry cigarette advertising as a matter of principle, notably *Reader's Digest, National Geographic,* the *New Yorker,* and *Good Housekeeping. Consumers' Reports* carries no advertising of any kind because of the need to maintain its independence and integrity, but remains consistently critical of the tobacco industry. Of the magazines aimed primarily at the women's market, *Seventeen* joins *Good Housekeeping* in having no truck with cigarette advertising, but the others derive millions of dollars per year from it, several more than $10 million a year apiece.[13]

ECONOMIC SANCTUARY

Advertising dollars have bought the cigarette companies protection against adverse discussion of the hazards of smoking in their chosen magazines. From 1982 to 1985, *Redbook* magazine did not publish a single article about smoking, but during the same period carried eleven articles about food and disease, ten about stress, and seven about skin care.[14] Also during 1982–1985 a general-interest magazine, *U.S. News and World Report,* carried eighteen articles about cancer, not one of which mentioned smoking. On October 8, 1984, *Time* published a special supplement on health, produced in cooperation with the American Academy of Family Physicians. The text contained no references to cigarette smoking. The academy stated that *Time* had removed all discussion of the health hazards of smoking, without the knowledge of the academy. That particular issue contained eight pages of cigarette advertisements.[15]

Of honorariums paid to United States senators and congressmen for speaking engagements during 1987, The Tobacco Institute paid $100,000, Brown and Williamson Tobacco Corporation (makers of Raleigh, Barclay, Kool, and Viceroy) paid $33,000, Philip Morris Inc. (makers of Benson & Hedges, Merit, Parliament, Marlboro, and Virginia Slims) and R. J. Reynolds Tobacco Company (makers of Camel, Salem, Winston, Vantage, More, and NOW) paid $29,000 each.[16] These payments constitute personal income to the recipient and are not contributions to campaign funds.

In April 1988, R. J. R. Nabisco Incorporated pulled out an $80 million account from the advertising agency that helped Northwest Airlines promote its new ban on smoking aboard all domestic flights. Said a vice president of the Tobacco Institute, "If we're attacked, we're not going to roll over and play dead. The sooner our adversaries, friendly or otherwise, learn that, the less difficulty they're going to find themselves in."[17]

Death In The West, a documentary film made by the British Broadcasting Company in 1976, interlaced old Marlboro commercials with interviews of company officials defending smoking, and with interviews of cowboys dying of lung cancer. The film was shown on London television to an estimated 12 million viewers in September 1976. Scheduled to be shown in the United States, it was forbidden temporarily when Philip Morris Inc. sued Thames Television and obtained a court order of prevention.[18] Since then, it has become available in this country. A similar film made in Australia, *A Tracheostomy for the Marlboro Man,* showed a cowboy type suffering from advanced emphysema, so severe that he required a permanent tracheostomy, continuing to smoke his cigarettes through the tracheostomy tube in his neck.

THE ADS ARE SELLING AN IMAGE

How is it possible for the cigarette companies to advertise a product known to have cumulative lethal effects? And to do it with such success? Observation of the advertisements in newspapers and magazines quickly suggests the answer: the ads are not selling the product itself, but are selling an image that has been built up around the product over the years. The image itself varies according to the group to which the sales pitch is directed. Many advertisements are directed at men; the image portrayed is of rugged supermen, so virile one wonders how they can stand it, puffing on their cigarettes. All in living color with backgrounds of the Golden West, mountains, forests, boots, saddles, and horse corrals. We have been conditioned to visualize the Marlboro man in such surroundings; so well conditioned, in fact, that we no longer visualize reality, the image that a habitual smoker actually presents. We are jarred sometimes, although we should know better, to see the would-be Marlboro man on the street, lighting up with a series of abrupt impatient gestures, then coughing and hawking onto the sidewalk.

The pitch is even more finely tuned in advertisements aimed at women. All those pictured are young and plainly in glowing good health; in many ads sexy, but invariably portrayed as strong-willed, independent, thinking for themselves. So doing, it says here, they are intensely appreciative of the new freedoms that young women enjoy, the freedom to smoke all they please apparently being one of the foremost. We have seen that cigarette manufacturers regard the women's market as their great opportunity, second within this country only to the opportunity of exposing children and teenagers of both sexes to the image of sophistication and maturity, an exposure which in time may cost them their lives.

Again, we have been so dazzled by the images that we have forgotten reality; and, sadly, it is anything but flattering. Reality was depicted in a poster distributed a few years ago by the American Cancer Society, captioned "SMOKING IS VERY GLAMOROUS!" A face peered from the poster, hair untidy, a cigarette dangling from the corner of its mouth. The picture, although most unflattering, brought a shock of instant recognition; each of us feels we know that person, and we see identical people every day on the street, or lighting up as they leave public buildings. No rebuttal of the glamour in cigarette advertising could be so effective as the unsparing eye, or ridicule. In Australia, a semi-underground group calling itself by an acronym in the Australian idiom, BUGA-UP, has taken to defacing cigarette billboards by making the message look stupid and fatuous.[19] (The actual name of the group was tortuously derived from the acronym, instead of the other way around: Billboard-Utilizing Graffitists Against Unhealthy Promotions!) The billboard guerrillas, using humor and ridicule as their allies, have gotten their message across much more effectively than if they had simply destroyed the advertisements.

Twenty

PROSPECTS FOR THE FUTURE

There was the Door to which I found no Key,
There was the Veil through which I could not see . . .

—Omar Khayyám, *Rubáiyát* (Fitzgerald
translation, Third Edition, 1872)

Whoso pulleth out this sword of this stone and anvil,
is rightwise born King of all England.

—Sir Thomas Malory, *Le Morte D'Arthur*
(1470)

POSSIBLE DURING OUR LIFETIMES?

Predicting the future is likely to be a foolhardy effort, even within the short span of five to ten years. In all probability, we should not attempt it. Arthur C. Clarke, master of science fiction, stated as a principle that "when an elderly and conservative scientist says a thing is impossible, he is almost certainly wrong." Then are any such predictions of value? Probably not. Having no guide but the past, we can consider the future only in the terms we understand. Any prophet who could foresee what improvements are to come in cancer treatment, surely would already hold in his or her hand the material for a Nobel Prize.

Surgical treatment of cancer is unlikely to progress much beyond its present state in terms of increasing the rates of cure, although it is likely that the risk of surgery will continue to decline through better understanding of anesthesia and postoperative care. Surgery continues to confound many past predictions that it could go no further, so that in our lifetimes we have seen such advances as organ transplantation, heart valve replacement, and coronary artery bypass. But the problem of cancer treatment is fundamentally a biologic one. Surgery may still refine somewhat its mechanical task of removing a primary tumor, but it cannot cope with the tendency of cancer to spread to other areas in the body, except in the rarest of cases. In particular, it cannot eradicate the invisible cells that may be spreading at the time of treatment. Surgery then could only improve its results in combination and partnership with the other disciplines.

For example, we have seen that the possibilities of cure by surgical treatment, as it exists today, would be greatly improved if earlier diagnosis of lung cancer became the norm. Improvements of this kind tend to come gradually and by evolution, and the presently available diagnostic tools have been tried but found to offer only limited chances of improvement. Entirely new diagnostic methods are likely to be needed, and it is difficult to see where they may come from, or what form they might take.

Improved methods of chemotherapy seem hopeful to many prognosticators. Could chemotherapy become potentially curative for most, or even many, of the common adult cancers? For the time being it seems most unlikely, if not impossible. A striking graph has tabulated each new anticancer drug according to the year in which it was introduced,[1] beginning slowly with the male and female hormones, then nitrogen mustard and methotrexate. The pace of new drug development quickened during the 1960s and 1970s, but has slowed again so that the curve has the form of half the bell-shaped curve of normal distribution. Does this mean that the discovery of new anticancer drugs is nearing an end, and that fewer if any will appear from now on? If so, we must write off chemotherapy as a potential means for real cancer control. I am referring to the potentially toxic and hazardous drugs that have monopolized the field of chemotherapy so far.

Only in relatively recent years, medicine has begun to build upon a secure basis of scientific understanding. Most of the cancer chemotherapy drugs in use today were discovered on an empirical basis, by means of trial and error. Few were developed rationally through understanding of the life processes. Many biochemists and cell biologists believe that eventually every programmed control mechanism and every chemical reaction within the body will be known. Presumably, it would then be possible to turn on and off the mechanisms responsible for malignant behavior of a cell, through chemical inducers or inhibitors. Such would be the crowning achievement of chemotherapy—the real magic bullet that could correct any aberration within the cells but would not injure normal cells.

Dr. Bill Hunter, disadvantaged by his role as a surgeon having to take care of sick people, and not a cell biologist with deep insight into life processes, still doubts that anything will come so easily. The question of "free lunch" unfortunately persists. The theory of the magic bullet requires distinct, exploitable differences in the chemical processes of malignant as opposed to normal cells, and hardly any such are known. The great German biochermist Otto Warburg (1883–1970), for example, studied utilization of oxygen by living cells and noted that cancer cells can derive a large part of their energy from breaking down glucose in the absence of oxygen, the process known as anaerobic glycolysis. The process is wasteful of energy, and injurious to normal cells after only a short time because of accumulation of metabolic acids which cannot be disposed of until oxygen is available. Nonetheless, cancer cells can use anaerobic metabolism with relative impunity. Hopes that such a difference could be exploited in treatment soon faded, after it was found that cancer cells also possess all the enzymes needed to fully metabolize sugars aerobically (with oxygen available), to water and carbon dioxide. Ability to use one or both metabolic pathways to extract energy from foodstuffs actually has made malignant cells more difficult to kill, not less; they can survive and multiply when normal cells are starving for oxygen. For the time being, then, cancer cells share all known life processes of normal cells, with the result that drugs toxic to them are injurious to normal cells also. Variable degrees of susceptibility to certain drugs make chemotherapy possible and sometimes dramatically helpful, but we have no access yet to any yes-or-no, 0-or-1 differences in susceptibility.

Will there be improved chemotherapy as an adjunct to surgery? Not unless chemotherapy itself improves dramatically; and in that case, the question may be whether surgery is necessary as a part of the treatment.

THE IMMUNE SYSTEM

Immunotherapy for cancer faces the same problem, a lack of clear-cut chemical or antigenic differences between normal and malignant cells of the same host. In the laboratory, cancers may be induced in small animals by injection of carcinogenic compounds, or by painting the compounds repeatedly on the skin. Under these circumstances doses are large and exposure to the carcinogens relatively intense, since the investigator wants tumors to develop quickly and in practically all animals. Such a rapid chemical induction of cancers has the effect of altering some of the characteristic proteins produced in the tumor, rendering the tumor anti-genically different and hence a potential target for immune reactions.

Strains of mice used in cancer research are highly inbred so that their genetic material is virtually identical between individuals, almost as between human identical twins. Called *syngeneic,* such animals readily accept skin or tissue grafts from each other, and even accept second grafts, which ordinarily would be rejected in accelerated fashion because the host had been sensitized or "immunized" by the first one. Within such strains, a cancer developing in one animal can be transplanted readily into another, and will behave in the recipient as though it were a new cancer. (Such acceptance of skin grafts or tumor grafts ordinarily is not possible outside the syngeneic or identical-twin [isogeneic] framework, because nonidentical tissue grafts are rejected. Rejection can be suppressed only by intensive treatment such as is given to organ-transplant recipients.)

Among the animals with tumors raised by carcinogenic chemicals, the original tumor will grow progressively and kill the host, because malignant tumors in some poorly understood way suppress and overcome the immune reactivity of their host. But other animals of the same strain can be sensitized against the new tumor with its altered proteins, so that when inoculated with live tumor tissue, they will reject it. The chemically induced tumor, transplanted into a sensitized host, is in biologic terms allogeneic or comparable to tissue from a noninbred animal. In a "naive" or nonsensitized syngeneic host, the tumor will keep on growing.

Findings of inducible rejection of syngeneic tumors seemed to offer brilliant promise that cancer could be controlled or eradicated in patients by immune means. Unfortunately, the promise was fallacious, for it turned out that immunization was not possible against spontaneously arising cancers. Rejectable tumors had been raised by abnormal means, therefore were bogus and not comparable to human cancer.[2] The spontaneously arising cancer has essentially the same pattern of proteins as does its host, is not antigenic to any significant degree, and does not appear to elicit any useful immune reaction in the host. No independently confirmed studies have shown that a human patient can be immunized against his spontaneous cancer.

In the case of lung cancer, since it is caused by chemical carcinogens in tobacco smoke, why does it not have the same immunogenicity? The laboratory animal models show that cancer induction by high-dose, short-term (weeks to several months) exposure to chemical carcinogens produces the greatest aberrations,[3] while long-term, low-dose administration may eventually induce cancers but with much less antigenic difference from the host. The twenty-year or greater lag period in most cases of lung cancer is by contrast a very long period of exposure to the carcinogen, and the resulting cancers' behavior and characteristics are indistinguishable from those of truly "spontaneous" tumors. (If indeed any such exist; those for which we cannot demonstrate a cause, we call spontaneous.)

Here, we must clarify an essential feature of the immune system as it has been understood in the past. The infant, animal or human, was thought to have been born with a clean slate, so to speak; not sensitized to anything, but already equipped with the mechanisms for recognition and "tolerance" of its own unique pattern of proteins, against which it would not react. Presented later with a foreign reactive substance or antigen, usually a distinctive protein from an infecting bacterium or virus, or injected foreign materials, the immune system develops the capacity to synthesize a specific chemical neutralizer of the antigen called an antibody. Upon later exposure to that same antigen, the antibody is formed very quickly and in large amounts, a phenomenon called immunologic memory. From this time on the individual is said to be sensitized against the antigen, common examples of which are the childhood vaccines against infectious diseases.

The essential feature of classical immunology was that immune reactivity did not occur until after exposure to or sensitization to the antigen. Without prior exposure, an individual would remain unreactive against a first exposure to it; while in the case of a spontaneously arising cancer, the host could not develop reactivity because the cancer cells presented only the same antigens that the host already recognized as "self." Truly foreign cells, such as those of a tissue graft or of a transplanted chemically induced cancer, are attacked and killed by certain white blood cells called lymphocytes, which first must have been sensitized against the foreign antigens. Plainly, the prospects for immune control of cancer were bleak.

This is not yet all of the story. Lymphocytes, the immunologically active cells, are not all the same but have several subgroups, each with its own functions within the immune system. Some, called T cells, depend on the thymus gland for their maturation and full development, while others, called B cells, develop largely in the bone marrow. Some T cells attack and kill foreign cells against which they have been sensitized, such as those of a tissue allograft, while others have a regulatory function and can suppress this killing under appropriate circumstances. Still others have a helper function to B cells in production of antibodies. But a few lymphocytes can attack and kill tumor cells or virus-infected cells, without the usual prior sensitization. Called "natural-killer cells," or NK cells, these enigmatic nonconformists belong to the group of immunologically active cells but do not follow the rules we associate with immunity.[4] What has primed them to kill only certain cells that are dangerous to the host? Not prior sensitization, so far as can be determined, because NK cells removed from a healthy person can kill cancer cells from other patients. (In this case, they have not been sensitized against the other person, either.) They do not attack or kill normal cells, but how they are able to recognize normal from malignant cells remains unknown. Why do NK cells not eradicate new cancers early, while they are small? This is a difficult question, and partial explanations may be that (1) there are not enough NK cells; (2) tumors probably exert suppressing mechanisms against them; and (3) tumors vary in their susceptibility to NK attack. Whatever the reasons during their early life history, it is clear that by the time tumors become identifiable, the NK system is inadequate to cope with them. The question arose whether NK cells could be strengthened, or stimulated to increase their numbers, so as to become more effective against an established cancer.

Various chemical signalers have been discovered, called *lymphokines*, which affect the movement and multiplication of lymphocytes; one of these was at first called T-cell growth factor, later interleukin-2, or IL-2 for short. Secreted in tiny amounts in the body under appropriate circumstances,[5] IL-2 now can be synthesized in large amounts through the technology of genetic engineering. Incubated outside the body with lymphocytes collected from a patient's blood, it is able to activate them as killer cells (called LAK, or lymphokine-activated killer cells) and stimulate them to increase greatly in number. Then, returned intravenously to the donor patient together with large continuing amounts of the stimulant, IL-2, these newly activated cells are indeed capable of inducing partial regression of the cancer in at least some patients, and complete regression in a very few.[6] Are LAK cells induced by this method different from naturally occurring NK cells? It is not entirely clear, since there are similarities as well as a few differences, but the induced LAK cells clearly can have a significant therapeutic effect on some cases of human cancer.

First reports of this new treatment method were hailed with great enthusiasm, but only further testing can confirm its usefulness. The method is enormously labor-intensive and involves great expense, paid for in the early studies by research grants. Only a few patients could be treated at a time. The large doses of IL-2 have considerable toxic effect, and fatalities from the treatment are possible. It remains to be seen whether the treatment can result in any cures, by itself or as an adjunct to surgery or radiation therapy. Chemotherapy may be less suited to combine with it, since today's chemotherapy has severe depressant effects on the white blood cells (including lymphocytes) and on the bone marrow which produces them.

Nevertheless, the LAK cell treatment is new and barely tried as yet. If further refinement and development are found to be possible, it may become a dramatic advance in cancer treatment. Is it immunotherapy? That is a matter of semantics, but it uses the cells active in the immune system. Many researchers speak of it as *adoptive immunotherapy*.

Brave New World?

Talk of cancer control by prevention is not exciting and dramatic as is discussion of possible new treatments, but our concern here is primarily with lung cancer. New curative treatments for lung cancer are not foreseeable with any assurance at all. Nevertheless this greatest killer among cancers could be prevented in 85 to 90 percent of cases, without any new discoveries or breakthroughs, and without any need for expensive high technology like that of the LAK-cell treatment. We know exactly how more than 100,000 cancer deaths per year in the United States could be prevented. What is more, the patients would not even need treatment.

Is there a wave of the future for the problem of lung cancer? Will it be in fundamental science? Proprietary and secret remedies? Freedom of choice in cancer treatment? Better than any, it would be to educate people in their own self-interest, and somehow to abolish their dependence upon the subconscious crutch, "It can' t happen to me."

Appendix A

Doubling Time as a Measure of Tumor Growth Rate

A Caliph, grateful to a courtier for services performed, summoned him before the court and asked him to name his own reward.

"Let a chess board be brought forward, O Caliph," replied the courtier. "Let a grain of wheat be placed on the first square, two on the next, four on the next, and so till the squares are filled. The grains of wheat shall be my reward."

Astonished that he should ask so little, the Caliph granted his request. (The total exceeds the entire world's wheat crop throughout all of human history.)

—Apocryphal

Some of the lung cancer patients discussed in this book survived only three to four months after the first diagnosis, in spite of treatment, while another survived nearly three years even though his disease could not be cured. Why should survival have varied over a tenfold range? Physicians speak of some cancers as being "highly malignant," meaning presumably that the patients have poor response to treatment and short survival. Could degree of malignant behavior be assessed during life? Tumor cell type is at least a partial guide; small-cell carcinoma in particular is known for its bleak prognosis. But even within the same cell type, individual tumors vary greatly in behavior. Finding of widespread metastases at the time of first diagnosis suggests, but does not prove, that the tumor is behaving with exceptional malignancy. (In this case we do not always know how long the primary tumor has been there.) Presumably rate of growth would correspond to degree of malignancy, but how exactly should it be measured? Physicians speak also of rapidly growing and slowly growing tumors, although such judgments are plainly subjective unless described in numbers.

A rounded, circumscribed tumor nodule in the periphery of the lung, the so-called coin lesion, offers the best opportunity for this kind of study. Two special features of the standard chest X-ray film are important here. First, each film bears a date and is a permanent record. Second, the film incorporates slight magnification of all body structures, since X-ray beams originate from a single point and expand outward in straight lines. Passing through the body and the tumor before reaching the X-ray film, they project onto the film a somewhat magnified image of the tumor. But the plain chest film is taken under standardized conditions, with projection in a postero-anterior (back-to-front) direction, and a distance of six feet between the X-ray source and the film cassette. (This is often called the 6–foot PA projection.) The patient stands facing the film cassette and against it, while the beam passes through the chest from back to front. If a denser nodule is present within the lung, its size is magnified slightly, but proportional magnification will always be uniform no matter when or where the film was taken. Some exceptions to this rule are portable or bedside films, taken at short tube-to-film distances and in an antero-posterior direction, plus a few others, but the exceptions can easily be excluded by inspection of the film.

Since magnification factors remain uniform on standard films, they may be disregarded for calculation of growth rate, and diameter of a rounded nodule may be measured directly from the film. Two chest films on the same patient, showing a measurable increase in diameter of the nodule, are sufficient to establish the rate of growth. Dates recorded on the films specify the time interval between observations.

HYPOTHESIS OF DOUBLING TIME

All living cells, including cancer cells, multiply by the process called *mitosis*, during which: (1) the cell manufactures a complete second copy of its chromosomes, (2) each full complement of chromosomes draws to oppposite poles of the cell, together with half of all the microscopic machinery of the cell, and (3) the cell divides into two. Mitosis may be described generically as a process of binary fission, meaning that one cell always splits into two.

If we assume that duration of the cell cycle, meaning the time interval between mitoses, remains fairly constant for a given malignant cell line, we could call it the *intermitotic time*. If we assume further that the malignant genotype is established by mutation in just one cell, then after successive divisions there will be two cells, four, eight, sixteen, thirty-two, sixty-four, and so on. After ten doublings, if no cells have been lost by cell death or other mishaps, the malignant cells will total 1,024 or approximately a thousand for our calculation in round numbers. After twenty doublings, they will total about a million or 10^6 cells; and if the cells average 10 microns in diameter, or about $1/100$ of a millimeter, the tiny collection of malignant cells will form an aggregate one millimeter (one twenty-fifth of an inch) in diameter. Little by little, the cell divisions have moved out of phase with each other in spite of approximately equal intermitotic times, so that the tumor does not suddenly double its volume all at once. Instead, with mitoses having gone gradually out of phase, the tumor appears to grow steadily in size. Its volume will be found to have doubled in a period equal to the approximate intermitotic time. After thirty doublings, the tumor will have 1,000 million or 10^9 cells and have a diameter of one centimeter, about four-tenths of an inch. From now on, still growing at an exponential rate, its size appears to increase with much greater rapidity. After forty doublings it will have grown to a large size, ten centimeters or four inches in diameter with a weight of about a kilogram (2.2 pounds), and containing a million million or 10^{12} cells.[1] (We used this size as the example of a far-advanced incurable tumor during discussion of chemotherapy in chapter 10.) By this time the patient is near death, and hardly any survive much longer with a cancer of this size. If we assume that the tumor kept on growing at the same rate, after only five more doublings (a total of forty-five), it would weigh about thirty-two kilograms (70 pounds) or almost half the body weight of an adult man (fig. A.1). This is impossible, and later on we shall take forty tumor doublings as approximately the limit of survival for the host.

So far, our discussion has been hypothetical, and we will consider how to test its validity. We should take note of some consequences that would follow if it is true. First, we saw that a tumor becomes possibly detectable at about the diameter of one centimeter, and that below this size it is in the subclinical or occult phase. The tumor reaches this size at about the thirtieth doubling. It follows that the cancer has already passed through three-quarters of its entire life history before it can even be detected, and in most cases it will have passed through much more than three-quarters. We have to understand that diagnosis and treatment are possible only

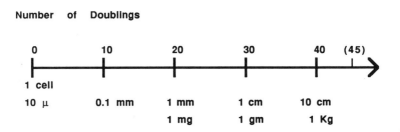

Figure A.1. Schematic diagram of the life history of a tumor, from the one-celled stage. (Source: Adapted from Ref. A–1.)

within the last one-quarter or less of the tumor's life span, putting the concept of "early" diagnosis and treatment into an entirely different light.

Second, the peculiarity of exponential growth (in this case, according to the powers of 2) is that as the tumor grows larger in gross or measurable size, it appears to grow ever faster. This is an illusion, but is the origin of the popular fallacy that an unsuccessful or exploratory operation "lights up the cancer and makes it spread all over the body." If the cancer could not be removed, it is already late; and from this time on its growth will appear to be progressively faster than the patient or family remember when they first became aware of it. They are likely to believe that it was stimulated by the operation to grow more rapidly.

MEASUREMENT AND CALCULATION

Diameter of a rounded nodule in the lung, seen on a chest X-ray, usually can be measured to about the nearest millimeter. (Remember that we will disregard the slight magnification factor, since it will remain uniform even though diameter is enlarging.) Then if we consider the nodule as a sphere, its volume may be calculated as $4/3 \pi r^3$, reducible to $4.18 r^3$. So the volume of a sphere varies as the cube of the radius. If the tumor's diameter (and radius) have doubled between measurements, its volume has increased by eight times, and the tumor has undergone three doublings (twice the volume, four times, eight times.) In approximate terms, the volume change with increments of diameter will run something like this:

Diameter	*No. of Doublings*	*Volume*
1.00x	0	1 y = (4.18) (0.5x)³
1.26x	1	2 y
1.59x	2	4 y
2.00x	3	8 y
2.52x	4	16 y
3.18x	5	32 y
4.00x	6	64 y

Assume, for example, that a tumor 4 centimeters in diameter is found on a patient's chest film. The patient remembers having had a previous X-ray just a year before, and when it can be obtained, the tumor is seen to be present but is only one centimeter in diameter; it is partially obscured by the collarbone shadow and was missed at the first reading. There have been six doublings in the transition from 1 to 4 cm. diameter (and the volume has increased by 64 times), so that the doubling time is easily calculated as two months.

How to calculate doubling time when the measurements are not such nicely rounded numbers? Let us try another example. A patient's chest film dated April 28, 1987, shows a rounded mass in the left upper lobe measuring approximately 4.2 centimeters in diameter. A previous film dated September 17, 1986, shows the nodule to measure 1.6 centimeters in the comparable diameter. The doubling time, DT, may be determined in either of two ways: first, by plotting the two measurements on semi-logarithmic graph paper in which the ordinate (vertical axis) represents tumor diameter (or radius) on a logarithmic scale, the abscissa or horizontal axis time on a simple scale. A moment's reflection will confirm that although tumor measurements were of diameter, tumor volume has been increasing as a logarithmic function and should be plotted accordingly. Now a straight line drawn through the two points plotted will intersect other lines which delineate a doubling in volume, and the time between these intersections may be read off the abscissa as the doubling time.[2] This method is an approximation at best, and cumbersome, but it reminds us that when tumor volume continues to grow according to geometric progression (as opposed to arithmetic), all measurements of diameter will continue to fall closely along this straight line (fig. A.2).

An approximation formula for calculation of doubling time has been devised:[3]

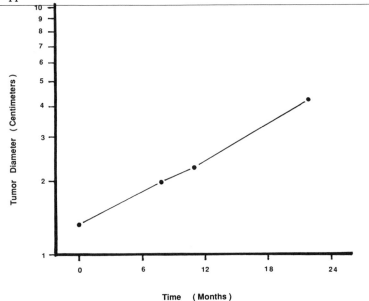

Time   (Months)

Figure A.2. Graphic pattern of progressive tumor growth, on a semi-logarithmic plot. Dots represent individual measurements of tumor diameter.

$$\text{Doubling time} \sim \frac{t}{10 \log (D_t/D_o)}$$

where t = time between measurements
      log = common logarithm (to the base 10)
      D_o = tumor diameter at first measurement
      D_t = tumor diameter at last measurement

This formula is accurate to within one-third of one percent, far less than the error of tumor measurements, so there is no need to resort to a precisely accurate formula devised by the same author. At the time it was published, the formula could be calculated easily on a slide rule, but now can also be determined with those pocket calculators which incorporate common logarithms. If we apply this formula to tumor measurements from the hypothetical patient, above, we find that interval between measurements was 224 days. D_t/D_o = 2.625, logarithm is 0.420, 10 times that is 4.2; 224 / 4.2 is 53.33 or a doubling time of about 53 days.

Of what practical value is this calculation? Doubling time gives us a number by which to characterize rate of tumor growth, although it can be calculated only for those tumors that are measurable as approximate spheres, and on which at least two observations are available showing a definite, measurable increase in diameter. Published studies indicate a median doubling time for all lung cancers in the range of about 80 to 90 days. Small cell carcinoma, the most malignant, frequently shows doubling times as short as 25–30 days; while some cases of bronchiolar-alveolar cell carcinoma have had doubling times as long as a year and a half. Calculation of doubling time emphasizes the wide range of growth rates even among tumors of the same cell type. The concept of exponential growth from the stage of a single cell has helped to define probability of cure in certain fairly rare malignancies of infancy, but these are outside the scope of our present discussion.

Patient survival could be predicted from two figures: (1) tumor diameter at first measurement, and (2) calculation of the number of doublings remaining before the tumor reaches the diameter of 10 centimeters, which we noted above as the approximate point of the 40th doubling and about the practical limit of survival.[4] Measured tumor diameter gives an index to the number of doublings so far, and therefore to how many remain before death; while if doubling time is known, the patient's approximate survival from that point can be predicted. Such an estimate of the tumor's natural history has proved to be fairly accurate, since treatment which fails to cure tends not to significantly prolong the patient's survival. In graphic form, most patients' survival falls closely along the "line of identity" between predicted and observed survival, while survival of a relatively small group of patients cured by surgery falls far above the predicted line (fig. A.3). Tumor spread or metastasis, we should recall, determines incurability, but thereafter the patient's survival is not improved by removal of the primary tumor.

Painstaking mathematical analyses of growth of transplantable tumors in small animals, principally mice, have concluded that all tumors show a declining growth rate with increasing age and size.[5] The "Gompertz equation" governing such a pattern expresses growth as initially exponential, but subject to a retarding factor whose effect increases with time, implying an eventual "horizontal asymptote" or arrest of growth. Suffice it to say that these equations are derived from a factitious biological system; practically all recorded observations of human cancer demonstrate continued exponential growth even over the maximum theoretically observable range of tenfold increase in diameter.

Does growth rate of a tumor correlate with its degree of malignancy? A

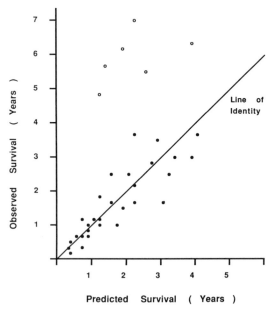

*Figure A.3. Correlation between predicted and observed patient survival from first measurement on X-ray, when the doubling time is known. Solid dots represent patients who died of their disease; Open dots represent the few patients cured by surgery. (*Source: *Adapted from Refs. A–3 and A–4.)*

small number of patients with primary lung cancer have had determination of doubling time before surgical treatment, plus recording of their survival thereafter.[6] Those with tumor doubling times over 150 days generally did well, while between 80 and 150 days a proportion were curable by surgery. Patients whose tumors doubled in less than 80 days did poorly. Similarly, prognosis has been examined for patients whose cancers elsewhere in the body had been eradicated, but who developed metastatic tumors in the lungs. (Cancers arising elsewhere often have their first spread to the lungs, because of the pattern of the two circulations, systemic and pulmonary. If the metastatic tumor in the lung is solitary, and there is no other spread, cure may be possible in some of these cases by surgical removal.) Pulmonary metastases, as they are called, are known to grow considerably faster in most cases than did the primary tumor, for reasons not known. Doubling time of 40 days was found to be an approximate dividing line between good and poor prognosis in those patients whose metastatic tumors were suited for surgical resection.[7]

Prediction of survival only on the basis of doubling time, wherever it can be measured, is of interest but is not necessarily the final answer. Very small tumors may still be curable by surgery even though they are growing rapidly. Tumor stage is a factor that can be defined in practically all cases, hence is more generally useful in determining prognosis.

A mathematician would say that doubling time is the reciprocal, the reverse if you will, of growth rate since a smaller number signifies faster growth and a larger number, slower growth. The objection is valid, but most of us can visualize a volume-doubling time much more easily than we can visualize a direct index of growth rate such as the coefficient of volume expansion with time. Most of us are not mathematicians.

Readers may have been confused by alternation of our discussions between doubling time on the one hand and logarithmic reduction of tumor burden on the other. Remember that we think of tumor growth in terms of powers of 2 because of the nature of cell division by mitosis. Tumor cell reduction by chemotherapy has no particular connection with powers of 2, and it is convenient to think of it in terms of powers of 10, the basis of common logarithms. The two methods come to a crossroads with each other, so to speak, at the level of approximately 1,000; this number is the factor for increase in the number of cells by each ten doublings, while at the same time cell reduction by a thousandfold is a reduction by "three logs."

Appendix B

HISTOLOGIC TYPES

For my part, whatever anguish of spirit it may cost, I am willing to know the whole truth—to know the worst and to provide for it.

**—Patrick Henry to the Virginia Convention
Richmond, March 23, 1775**

I have alluded several times in the text and glossary to the different histologic types, or cell types, of lung cancer. These can affect the patient's prognosis, because of variation between types in rate of growth, tendency to metastasize early versus late, to recur after treatment, or in other manifestations of malignant behavior. Cell type is identified by the pathologist during his examination of stained microscopic sections from the tumor. The pathologist often may consult with colleagues regarding the verdict, since no one person's diagnosis is always secure and automatic but involves a good deal of interpretation; in very difficult cases slides may be sent to pathologists at other medical centers for further consultation. Such consultation is needed especially when much depends on the acccuracy of diagnosis. The tissue being examined may have been obtained from a biopsy, from the diseased organ removed at operation, or sometimes even from a tumor found at autopsy.

The major primary carcinomas of the lung of high malignancy, the "lung cancers" of which we have been speaking in this book, are four in number:[1]

SQUAMOUS CELL CARCINOMA
These arise from flattened squamous cells similar to those of the epidermis or the mucous membranes of the mouth. Squamous epithelium does not occur naturally in the lung or bronchial tubes, but can develop

from the normal epithelium of the respiratory tract by a process called metaplasia ("growth in a different form") which results from exposure to carcinogens such as cigarette smoke. With continued exposure, metaplasia can proceed to formation of obvious cancer. Most textbooks still say that squamous cell carcinoma is the commonest type of lung cancer, but several reviews find that adenocarcinoma has been more common in recent years.[2] Reasons for this apparent change in frequency remain obscure, but possibly are related to slowly changing criteria for histologic diagnosis.

Squamous cell carcinoma, when it is found to be localized at the time of diagnosis, tends to have somewhat better prognosis for surgical cure than do the other types, and less tendency toward early microscopic spread. This difference is only relative, and many cases of squamous cell carcinoma show highly malignant behavior. Those tumors called "anaplastic" or "poorly differentiated" squamous carcinoma tend to be more malignant in behavior than those identified as "well differentiated." The tumor is moderately sensitive to radiation therapy, but unfortunately almost insensitive to chemotherapy. Ninety-two to 96 percent of cases have a strong association with smoking history. Squamous cell carcinoma tends to be second in frequency to small cell carcinoma among persons exposed to radon inhalation; but inexplicably, in some areas in which miners are exposed to radon, squamous carcinoma has been almost the sole type.[3]

ADENOCARCINOMA OF THE LUNG

I have noted in the glossary that the prefix "adeno-" signifies a relationship to glands; thus adenocarcinoma arises from glandular structures and preserves in its microscopic architecture the characteristic sac-shaped patterns of glandular cells. (Childhood adenoids = like or similar to glands, but not actually glands; these are collections of lymphatic tissue, as are tonsils, in the back of the nasal cavity.) In the lining of the bronchial tree are many bronchial mucus glands, the probable sites of origin of bronchial adenocarcinoma.

Adenocarcinoma, along with large-cell undifferentiated carcinoma, tends on the average to show somewhat more malignant behavior than does squamous cell carcinoma. We have noted previously that in recent years it has become the commonest type of lung cancer, for reasons that are not clear. Thirty years ago, and more, it was often called the "women's lung cancer" because of the supposition that it bore no relation to smoking history, and that lung cancer seldom if ever afflicted women. Neither of these suppositions is true any longer; in one study 89 percent of new patients with adenocarcinoma of the lung had been cigarette smokers.[4] But among the few nonsmokers who develop lung cancer, adenocarcinoma remains the commonest type. Adenocarcinoma also is moderately responsive to radiation treatment, but only poorly responsive to chemotherapy.

LARGE-CELL UNDIFFERENTIATED CARCINOMA

This type comprises a more heterogeneous group of tumors, in histologic appearance as well as clinical behavior. Some pathologists concede that tumors are assigned to this group not because they are similar to each other, but because they lack specific features that characterize the other types. In microscopic sections, these tumors are composed of fairly large cells, irregular in size and shape, pattern of the nucleus, and so on. The great majority are associated with a smoking history. Their behavior tends to be distinctly more malignant than that of squamous cell carcinoma, and chances of cure tend to be poorer. These tumors are possibly less responsive than the other types to radiation, and practically unresponsive to chemotherapy.

SMALL-CELL UNDIFFERENTIATED CARCINOMA

This type, also known as small-cell carcinoma, is the fastest-growing and the most malignant of this group of tumors. Its behavior and prognosis are so different from the others that most papers and research studies on lung cancer divide all tumors into two groups, small-cell and non-small-cell carcinomas. Small-cell carcinoma has two known causes, smoking and radon inhalation. We need to remember that this type cannot be treated with hope of cure by surgery alone, that it practically always is spreading by the time of first diagnosis, is sensitive to both radiation therapy and combination chemotherapy, and usually is treated by both these methods. Practically all patients show response to treatment, and have prolongation of survival, but few are cured.

VARIANT AND NONSMOKING-RELATED MALIGNANCIES

Certain other tumor types need to be mentioned for the sake of completeness, but do not compare in degree of malignancy to the four types listed above. These types are relatively uncommon, do not bear any clear relation to smoking history, and ordinarily are not included in discussions of "lung cancer" or "primary bronchogenic carcinoma" because of the differences in their behavior as well as causation.

BRONCHIOLAR OR ALVEOLAR-CELL CARCINOMA

This is a fairly uncommon tumor, somewhat similar to adenocarcinoma in histologic appearance, but arising from the lining cells of the air sacs and terminal passageways, far out in the periphery of the lung. Paradoxically, it may appear clinically in one of two ways: first and more commonly, with an appearance on X-ray films suggestive of slowly progressive diffuse fibrosis or scarring of the previously clear lung tissue, gradually spreading and often bilateral (involving both lungs) by the time of diagnosis. Diagnosis generally requires direct surgical biopsy of the lung, but in this mode of presentation surgery is of no use as treatment. No effective treatment is possible at this stage except for a slight possibility of temporary response to chemotherapy; even so, progression of the disease is very slow and often goes on for several years. The second and more favorable presentation, occurring in a minority of cases, is as an asymptomatic solitary nodule (coin lesion) in the periphery of the lung. In this presentation, the tumor has an unusually good prognosis if treated surgically. In either form, growth of this tumor tends to be extremely slow.

Researchers have been intrigued by the possible multicentric origin (arising at multiple sites) of this tumor, as well as by its microscopic similarity to an infectious disease of sheep, malignant pulmonary adenomatosis or, as it is known in the Afrikaans language of South Africa, "*jaagziekte*." This is a virus infection which spreads between animals, producing multiple malignant tumors in the lungs which cause the death of the animal. Unfortunately, no secure evidence has yet appeared that human bronchiolar-alveolar-cell carcinoma is caused by a virus, and its similarity to the infectious disease of sheep may simply be coincidental.

BRONCHIAL ADENOMAS

A group of tumors known collectively as Bronchial adenomas must be included here because they are actually low-grade malignancies, but, again, not comparable to the true bronchogenic carcinomas. Their name is a misnomer since the word *adenoma* means a benign tumor of glandular origin. Common usage unfortunately has perpetuated the name. None of these tumors bear any relation to smoking history.

1. Carcinoid tumors of the bronchus tend to appear in the age range of the twenties and thirties, are located mostly in large bronchi so that almost all can be seen through a bronchoscope, and produce symptoms either as a result of infection beyond a partially obstructed bronchus, or of bleeding with resultant hemoptysis. They grow slowly and are slow to spread, so that the great majority are curable by surgical removal. A few tumors, especially those showing "atypical histology," a disorganized microscopic pattern, are more malignant in behavior and may spread or metastasize widely. The word carcinoid means similar to carcinoma (in microscopic appearance), but not the same as.

2. Adenocystic carcinomas are properly named as malignancies, but are very slow growing and late to metastasize. Known in former years as cylindromas, they occur primarily in the trachea, or "windpipe," do not bleed, and produce symptoms of very slowly progressive airway obstruction. Location in the trachea usually eliminates any possibility of surgical treatment for cure. Effective palliation over a period of years has often been possible by widening the airway passage at intervals with biopsy forceps, or a laser beam, through a rigid bronchoscope; and some cases have responded to cobalt radiotherapy.

3. Muco-epidermoid tumors of the bronchi also are low-grade malignancies, slow growing, usually producing symptoms by bronchial obstruction and resulting infection in the area of lung distal to the tumor. They do not tend to bleed. Most can be located through the bronchoscope, and most are curable by surgical excision.

LYMPHOMAS

These may be primarily located in the lung, and often are not diagnosed until the time of thoracotomy. In the present day, surgery has limited if any usefulness in their treatment; but if involvement is limited to a lobe or less, surgery can induce complete remission immediately and thus benefit subsequent definitive treatment by chemotherapy.

Appendix C

CHEST X-RAYS AND COMPUTERIZED TOMOGRAPHY

(In possible encounters with a culturally superior race): Any sufficiently advanced technology will be indistinguishable from magic.

—Arthur C. Clarke (1917–)

Diagnostic X-ray studies of the human body have limitations to their usefulness. Unfortunately they cannot show "everything that's inside you" as a popular misconception holds, but instead show only a pattern of shadows cast by the X-ray beam after passing through tissues of differing density. Bones, because of their mineral content, have the highest density and can be shown clearly without any difficulty. The "soft tissues"— muscles, internal organs, brain, and so on, tend to be of fairly uniform density and to cast continuous shadow, within which the separate structures cannot be distinguished except by the introduction of contrast materials. Body fat has lower density than the other soft tissues and often can help to delineate other structures that it surrounds or separates. ("Density" in this context refers to the degree to which a tissue absorbs or partially blocks the passage of X-ray beams through it. High-density materials such as bone will block passage of the rays to a much greater extent than will soft tissues such as muscle, or very low-density tissues such as fat.) Air has the lowest density of all, so that tissues containing air appear the most lucent on an X-ray film, having allowed passage of the beams with hardly any obstruction at all.

What tissues of the body contain air? Scattered collections of air are present normally in the stomach and throughout the intestinal tract. When the intestine becomes obstructed, as from adhesions, blockage by tumor, or other factors, air accumulates behind the obstruction and distends the intestine in a characteristic manner that can be seen on plain X-ray films, helping greatly in the diagnosis. But the primary organs of the body that contain air are the lungs; after all, their function is one of air and gas exchange with the environment. So the lungs are characteristically lucent on plain chest X-rays, and their extent is immediately obvious. Another feature is that the lungs are traversed by many fine structures denser than air, namely the pulmonary artery branches, pulmonary vein branches, the walls of the large and smaller bronchi, and even the fissures between lobes, so that the lungs' characteristic appearance includes multiple strands and cobwebby shadows extending from the hilum out through the air-containing lung tissue. A notable X-ray change occurs when air has gotten into the pleural space, letting the lung collapse from its own inherent elasticity, a situation called *pneumothorax* from the Greek for "air in the chest". The chest filled with air alone shows an appearance of absolutely clear lucency, without the lung's fine vascular and bronchial shadows.

Conversely, if the main bronchus to the lung has been obstructed, as by a tumor, air in the lung beyond that point will be rapidly absorbed leaving the appearance of atelectasis, airless collapse. Without air, the lung tissue involved by atelectasis shows contraction, or loss of volume, and density similar to that of solid tissue such as muscle or liver. A tumor in the lung of visible size, being made up of solid tissue, will be denser than the surrounding lung and will stand out as a solid density (unless of course the tumor has caused atelectasis, which can obscure its outlines). A peripheral nodule or coin lesion will stand out within the air-containing lung and be measurable.

"Reading" X-ray films, therefore, involves considerable interpretation of the patterns of density of shadows on the film and changes that may have occurred. Thorough knowledge of anatomy is a necessary background, plus large accumulated experience and familiarity with the types of change that may be associated with various disease processes. It should follow that persons without a medical background are not in a position to dispute interpretation of X-ray films with a radiologist. If a patient or family have any doubt about the reading, they are free to ask for other or additional opinions, but in no way should they rely upon their own.

X-RAY FILMS OF THE CHEST

Standard size for films of the adult chest is fourteen by seventeen inches. Two films are usually taken, in the antero-posterior (AP) or frontal projection, and the lateral projection. Each has advantages and disadvantages for visualization of structures within the chest, but they complement each other. The X-ray film is a negative transparency, similar to negatives of black-and-white camera film, recording greater exposure to the rays as black tones and greater absorption of the rays by tissue such as bone as light tones. Films are read with the help of transillumination on an X-ray view box, a glass panel lighted from behind. A large viewing box with many lighted panels allows review of numerous films in time sequence, or in side-by-side comparison.

THE FRONTAL CHEST FILM

By convention, chest films are viewed as though the examiner were facing the person being examined, so that the right side of the patient's body in the film is to the examiner's left (fig. C.1). The bones are the structures of greatest density and show as light shades in this negative film; first, the vertebrae or bones of the spinal column, which run up the midline of the body in this view. Twelve are in the area of the chest and are called thoracic vertebrae. A pair of ribs, a right and a left, are attached to each thoracic vertebra and run around the sides of the chest, forming a bony cage for the chest cavity. The sternum, or breast-bone, does not show well in the frontal projection since its image is projected over the spinal column and the mediastinal density, but it can be seen in the lateral projection. Near the upper border of the chest, the clavicles or collarbones act as braces between the sternum and the bones of the shoulder joint. The two shoulder joints, each with a shallow ball-and-socket configuration, are seen on all chest films but not in the best of detail.

The lungs occupy the two large areas of relative clarity (that is, dark tones in the negative film) within the smooth curves of the rib cage and on either side of the vertical midline density (light tones) of the mediastinum. The lowermost border of each lung is marked by the smooth, rounded dense contour of the diaphragm, dense because immediately under it are the large organs of the abdomen. At this level these are principally the liver, spleen, and stomach; liver and spleen are uniformly of solid-tissue density while a pocket or large bubble of air generally can be seen within the stomach.

The right lung is somewhat larger than the left, the latter being reduced in size because of the space occupied by the heart. At about the midpoint of the chest in a top-to-bottom direction, along the margin between lung and mediastinum, a bunching together of the strandlike

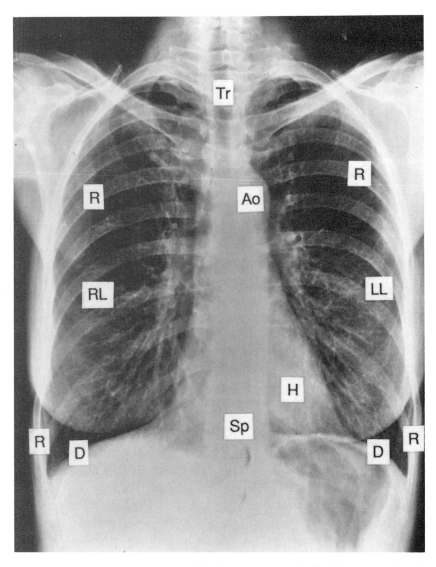

Figure C.1. Frontal plain film of the chest ("6-foot PA film") on a patient in complete remission after treatment for small-cell carcinoma of the lung, hence by definition an essentially normal film. RL, right lung; LL, left lung; R, ribs; D, diaphragm; H, heart; Sp, spinal column, within the mediastinal shadow; Ao, aorta, the great artery leaving the heart, also within the mediastinal shadow; Tr, air column of the trachea, passing from the neck down into the mediastinum.

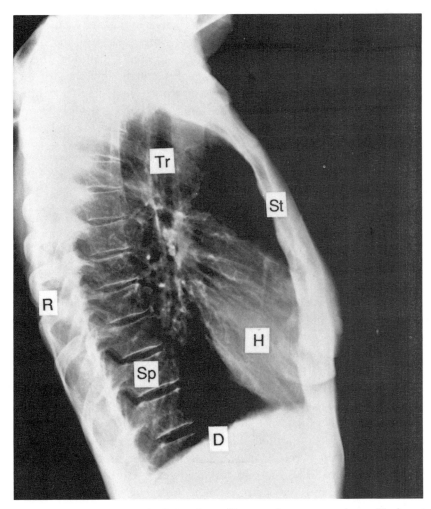

Figure C.2. Right lateral plain chest film on the same patient. H, heart shadow; R, ribs seen best posteriorly; D, diaphragm; Sp, spinal column; St, sternum or breast-bone; Tr, air column of the trachea.

shadows within the lung marks the hilum or root of the lung on each side. The main bronchus, pulmonary artery, and two pulmonary veins enter or leave the lung at the hilum. Figures C.1 and C.2 are chest films of a patient who achieved complete remission after treatment for small-cell carcinoma of the lung; hence by definition they show no residual signs of the tumor. The two lungs in this particular film are clear, except for diffuse changes resulting from chronic smoking; these changes would be difficult to explain but are immediately obvious to the eye of a radiologist. X-ray shadow of the mediastinum contains the shadows of the vertebral column, the heart, and the mediastinal structures including the great blood vessels. The smooth dense bulge of the mediastinal density toward the patient's left (viewer's right) in the frontal view, just above the diaphragm, is the heart shadow. Several of the contours of this heart shadow, in both the frontal and lateral projections, may be indicators of enlargement of individual chambers of the heart.

THE LATERAL CHEST FILM

While the lateral chest film is being taken, the patient's arms must be raised overhead so that the large bones in the upper arm do not obscure details within the chest. In the lateral projection the images of right and left lungs and mediastinum all are superimposed, and if a mass is present in one lung, we can not tell from this one film whether it is on the right or left side. We can tell, however, whether it is located anteriorly or posteriorly within the lung, or within the mediastinum in the case of a mediastinal mass. (The frontal film could not have told us this.)

Looking at the lateral film (fig. C.2), we should once more check the bony structures of the chest first. The bones of the spine, vertebrae, are seen forming a slightly curved vertical column about three-quarters of the way back in the chest. The ribs may be seen curving around the chest in a somewhat downward direction from back to front, but are not prominent in this projection. The sternum, or breastbone, is the farthest forward, also not a very dense bone and not seen prominently on ordinary chest films. The more or less oval shadow of the heart lies anteriorly, just behind the sternum. The lungs again occupy the large, relatively clear area inside the ribs and above the diaphragm; two separate contours of the diaphragm are often seen, representing the right and left sides, with uniform solid-tissue density below. The lungs extend posteriorly beyond the spinal column, since the latter protrudes forward into the chest, and the lungs also extend anteriorly to the very front of the chest. In this lateral view, the uppermost or apical portions of both lungs are obscured by the relatively heavy shadows of the shoulders. The hilum of each lung is located just about in the center of the lung in this view, and the two hilums are usually superimposed upon each other. The *fissures* which I have discussed as separating lobes often can be seen in the lateral film as fine lines of increased density, the major fissure running obliquely from the upper-posterior area of the lung down to the lower-anterior corner. Any masses located within the mediastinum may not be visible on lateral films unless they protrude right or left into the lungs. When fluid is present within the chest cavity (none is present here), it naturally pools at the bottom of the chest while the patient is in the erect position, and thus may be seen as solid density obscuring the lowermost portion of the aerated lung. One other detail is of some interest: the two sides of the chest, although superimposed in this view, appear to be of somewhat different size. We should remember that one side of the chest was closer to the X-ray beam source, and farther from the film, than was the other side when the film was exposed. As a result, the lung and rib cage farther from the film will be somewhat magnified as compared to the nearer. In the frontal projection, the slight factor of magnification ordinarily is equal for both sides of the chest.

A COIN LESION IN THE LUNG

Figures C.3 and C.4 are the frontal and lateral chest films of a fifty-eight-year-old man, a heavy smoker since his teens. The patient could not remember when he had previously had a chest X-ray taken. Let us review the frontal film first, C.3. The bony structures of the chest show no obvious abnormalities. The heart shadow is of normal size and configuration, as are the diaphragmatic contours on each side. The rib cage flares outward noticeably in the lower one-third or so of the chest, a collateral sign of long-standing emphysema. Below the left diaphragm, gas bubbles are seen in the stomach and probably also in the colon or large intestine. We see the air column of the trachea coming down from the neck into the upper mediastinum. The mediastinal shadow is approximately in the midline, overlying the vertebral column. Both lungs are fully aerated and show no evidence of atelectasis or loss of volume. The hilar shadows on both sides are fairly prominent, as is common in smokers of this age, and there is a calcified density within the left hilum, probably the residual of an old chronic infection.

In about the midportion of the right lung field (on the viewer's left) there is an approximately round, fairly well-defined shadow of increased density, marked by the arrow. We take this to be solid tissue because its density is clearly greater than that of the aerated lung surrounding it. There are no special or unusual features to its appearance. No evidence of calcification can be seen within it, nor any cavitation. No satellite

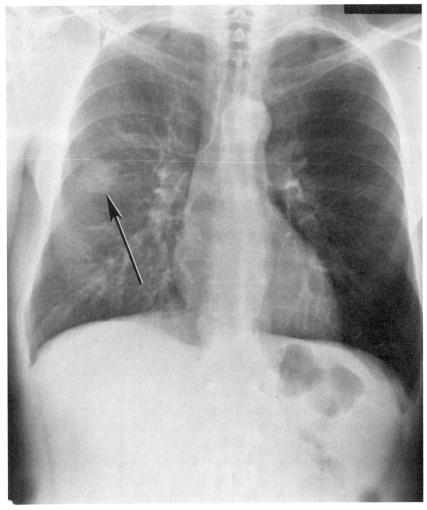

Figure C.3. Frontal plain chest film showing a rounded circumscribed density (arrow) in the periphery of the right lung.

nodules are present, nor infiltrate in the surrounding lung suggestive of infection or inflammation.

Now we must study and compare the lateral film, figure C.4. We are looking at it as though at the right side of the patient's chest. The chest is distinctly enlarged in the antero-posterior, or A-P, diameter, and the contours of the diaphragm are definitely flatter, less curved, than nor-

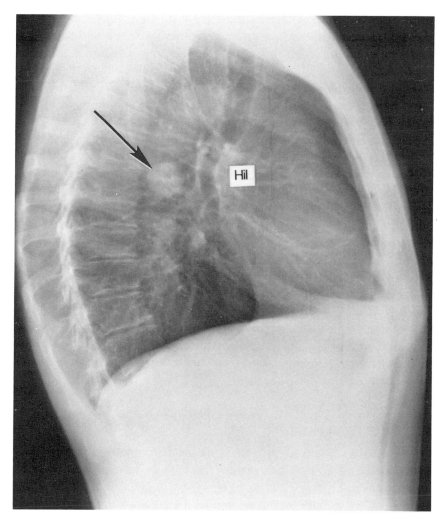

Figure C.4. Right lateral plain chest film on the same patient, again showing the "coin lesion" (arrow). Hil, hilar shadows of the two lungs, superimposed.

mally. Both these changes are cardinal signs of long-standing emphysema, the former often referred to as the "barrel chest" configuration. We see the cardiac silhouette in the lateral view, above the diaphragm and up forward in the chest, and the arch of the aorta extending above it. The tracheal air column also is seen coming down to its point of division within the overlapping hilar shadows, just about in the center of the chest. The rounded density again is seen within the lung tissue, somewhat posterior to the hilum in this·projection. The major fissure is not definitely visible in this film, and, as a result, we cannot say with certainty whether the density is located within the right upper lobe or the right lower lobe. (It is located too far posteriorly to be within the right middle lobe.) The nodule appears to be slightly below the usual location of the fissure, and our estimate would be that it is within the lower lobe.

A radiologist's summary of this interpretation might read as follows: "Films of the chest show changes of long standing emphysema and evidence of long continued smoking. Contours of the heart and great vessels are within normal limits for a patient of this age. A rounded, circumscribed density measuring approximately 2.5 centimeters in diameter is located within the right lung, probably within the right lower lobe. No old films are available for comparison. As far as can be determined, this appears to be a new lesion in a long-time smoker. Its radiographic appearance is compatible with a primary carcinoma of the lung."

The tumor proved to be an apparently localized small-cell carcinoma of the lung. No involved lymph nodes were present. The patient received the full course of combination chemotherapy following lobectomy, plus prophylactic radiation therapy to the brain. Unfortunately, the tumor subsequently recurred in the liver.

A REVIEW OF SERIAL FILMS

Figures C.5, C.6, and C.7 are all in the frontal projection; lateral films taken on the same days are omitted here, since frontal films serve to demonstrate the finding. Figure C.6 is dated January 20, 1988. The patient had seen his physician on that day, complaining of malaise, weakness, increased cough which recently had been productive of small flecks of blood, and increased shortness of breath. He had been a long-time heavy smoker. His last previous chest X-ray had been taken in June 1986 (fig. C.5). The patient lived at a distance from the medical center to which his physician wished to refer him and was reluctant to make the trip. His reluctance and other factors resulted in a delay of two and a half months before he actually was admitted there for diagnosis and treatment; figure C.7 is his chest film on the day of admission, April 6, 1988.

The old film from 1986 shows no particular abnormalities except for slightly prominent hilar shadows, compatible with late middle age and

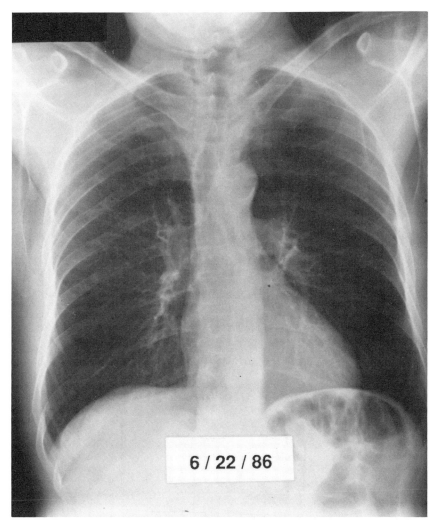

Figure C.5. Last normal chest film, June 1986, on the same patient shown in the next two figures. Film shows changes resulting from chronic smoking, but no sign of a tumor.

long-continued smoking. On the film of January 1988, a poorly defined mass density is apparent in the left lung, located at the lower part of the hilum. It is a new lesion, new within two and a half years at most, and its appearance is entirely consistent with primary cancer of the lung. The third film, after the subsequent delay, shows that the mass has grown

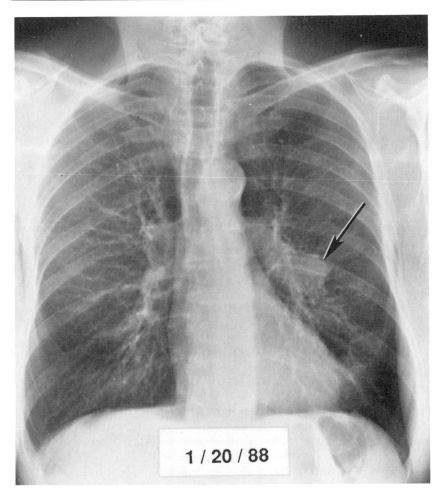

Figure C.6. Same patient; chest film after the onset of symptoms, January 1988. Film shows a poorly defined mass in the lower pole of the left hilum (arrow).

considerably in the interim. Its contour is even less well-defined than before. Accurate measurement of its diameter is not really possible, and only the roughest estimate could be made of the doubling time. Biopsy showed the tumor to be a poorly differentiated squamous cell carcinoma, and the patient underwent left pneumonectomy, removal of the entire left lung. The outcome is not yet determined, but it seems likely that the tumor's rapid growth will be an adverse factor in his prognosis.

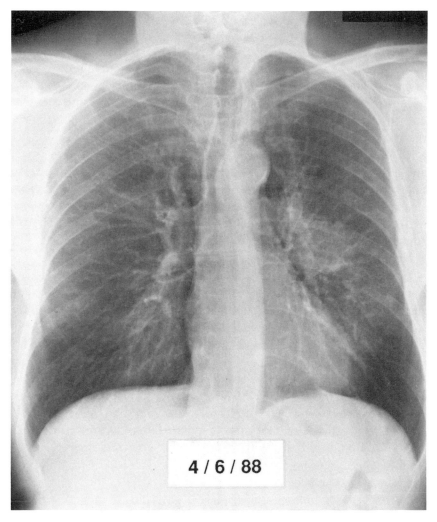

4 / 6 / 88

Figure C.7. Same patient; chest film at time of admission to the hospital, after more than two months' delay. The tumor mass has enlarged significantly in the interim.

COMPUTERIZED TOMOGRAPHIC SCANNING OF THE CHEST

A fairly new radiographic study technique is known as computerized tomographic, or CT, scanning. (The popular term "CAT" scanning confuses terminology and obscures understanding of the process; we would do better to avoid it.) Film images produced by CT scanning offer an entirely different way of looking at the body. While conventional X-ray films "look" one way through an area of the body (such as the chest) from back to front, or from side to side, the CT record resembles a succession of cross-sectional cuts through the body. The serial images are reviewed in numerical sequence, allowing the examiner to visualize internal anatomy from top to bottom of the body area being examined. It is as though the imaginary body were cut entirely into transverse slices 1 centimeter thick, as a salami is cut, beginning at the top of the head. Then the slices are laid out in rows, in order, so that they may be inspected in a serial manner. Going from one to the next, the examiner can pick out all body structures as they appear and then disappear from the cross-sections.

To undergo this examination, the patient lies supine on a narrow stretcher, arms raised over the head if the chest is to be examined. The stretcher is positioned appropriately inside a doughnut-shaped structure which closely surrounds the patient's body. The doughnut contains an X-ray beam source on one side of the circle, a sensitive receiving screen on the opposite side, and a mechanical apparatus which rotates the two in a full circle around the chest while the X-ray beam is being transmitted. Electrical signals produced by X-ray beams falling on the screen are fed constantly into a computer; the signals received during a full rotation are synthesized into a single cross-sectional image of the body at that level. The apparatus then moves downward one centimeter and repeats the process. Successive images are recorded on X-ray film, again in black-and-white negative form but much reduced in size. Also recorded is a miniature frontal film of the chest, with transverse lines drawn across it by the computer, marking the level at which each successive transverse body image was made.

By convention, images are displayed and read as though with the patient supine, the examiner looking at the underside of the body slice. As a result, the right side of the patient's body is to the examiner's left, and vice versa. And since the radiographic density of the air-containing lungs is so much less than that of the body's solid tissues, the images are displayed by the computer at two density settings: one at lung density so as to show fine detail within the lung, but no detail elsewhere; the other at mediastinal density settings, to show detail in the solid tissues.

Figures C.8 and C.9 are of two images, at the same body level, on the patient whose plain chest film we have seen in figure C.7. The first image, C.8, is shown at the dark or mediastinal density settings, so that the lungs

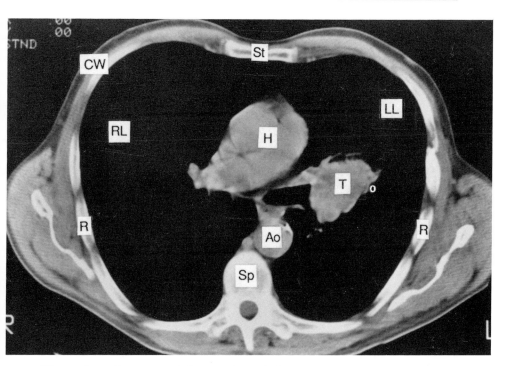

Figure C.8. Transverse CT image through the chest, at "mediastinal density" settings; same patient and same time as the chest film in Figure C.6. Large poorly defined tumor mass in area of the left hilum. RL, right lung; LL, left lung; CW, chest wall; R, ribs; St, sternum or "breastbone"; H, heart; T, tumor; Ao, aorta; Sp, spinal column (one of the vertebrae) in transverse section.

appear entirely black (overexposed) without any visible detail. Outside the lungs, the structures of the chest wall are seen in detail: the vertebra or bone of the spinal column with its neural canal enclosing the spinal cord; several ribs in oblique section; the scapulas, or shoulder-blades, embedded in the heavy shoulder muscles; and the sternum or breastbone anteriorly. (Note the markers of right and left sides.) Within the chest can be seen the heart shadow anteriorly, with some detail of its chambers, and the aorta posteriorly, adjacent to the vertebra. In the hilum of the patient's left lung (to the viewer's right) is the large irregular mass of the tumor.

Figure C.9, at the lung-density settings which can be thought of as

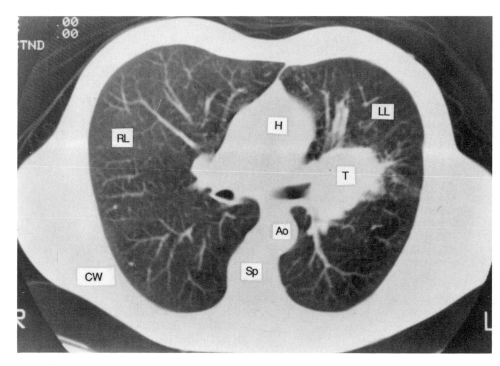

Figure C.9. Same patient, same examination, same transverse image, but shown at the "lung density" settings. Fine detail is now visible throughout the lungs. RL, right lung; LL, left lung; CW, chest wall; H, heart; T, tumor; Ao, aorta; Sp, Spinal column, obscured within the body wall.

comparable to an underexposed photograph, reveals no detail within the chest wall. The heart silhouette and the tumor mass can be seen but again without detail, since their density is that of solid tissue. Fine detail is visible throughout the two lungs; the branching twiglike structures are the small branches of the pulmonary arteries and veins. Two dark spots, one just each side of the midline in about the center of the chest, are the right and left main bronchi. Both are dark (radio-lucent) even in this underexposed film, because they contain air only. The important point is that no evidence of other, small, tumors can be seen.

Finally, figure C.10 shows a single image, at the lung density settings, of the same patient whose plain chest films were shown in figures C.3 and C.4. Again, fine detail is seen within the lungs, but not within the heart shadow or the chest wall. Right and left main bronchi may be seen, with a

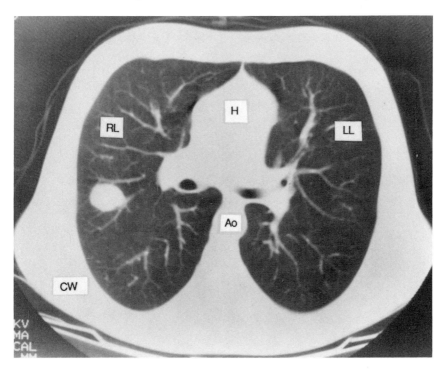

Figure C.10. Transverse CT image, number 13, on the same patient shown in figures C.3 and C.4; at the "lung density" settings. The tumor is in the right mid-lung field, not marked. RL, right lung; LL, left lung; CW, chest wall; H, heart shadow; Ao, shadow of the aorta, obscured within the mediastinal density.

second, more lateral, image of the smaller left upper lobe bronchus. The tumor is plainly seen within the right midlung field; but contrary to our previous impression from the plain chest films C.3 and C.4, this CT image demonstrates that the tumor actually is located within the right upper lobe. Slightly below the tumor, a band of relative clarity (absence of vessel shadows) runs obliquely from the hilum out to the chest wall, and it can be identified from study of the serial images as the location of the major fissure. The portion of lung tissue with its fine blood vessels posterior to that relatively clear band represents the apex of the right lower lobe, while the portion of lung lateral and anterior to it is the right upper lobe. (The tumor indeed was found at the operation to be confined within the right upper lobe.) Such subtle findings demonstrate the value of CT scanning as a complement to plain chest X-rays.

Notes

CHAPTER 1. IMPRINTING

1. E. L. Wynder and E. A. Graham, Tobacco smoking as a possible etiologic factor in bronchiogenic carcinoma: A study of six hundred and eighty-four proved cases. *Journal of the American Medical Association* 1950; 143: 329–336. (Dr. Wynder was a medical student at Washington University in St. Louis at the time of this report; Dr. Graham was professor and chairman of the Department of Surgery. Dr. Graham, among his many other accomplishments, had been the first to successfully remove a patient's entire lung as treatment for cancer, in 1933.)
2. *Smoking and Health*. Report of the Advisory Committee to the Surgeon General of the Public Health Service. Washington, D. C.: U. S. Department of Health, Education, and Welfare, 1964.
3. *The Health Consequences of Smoking: Smoking and Cancer*. A Report of the Surgeon General. Publication DHHS (PHS) 82–50179. Washington, D. C.: U. S. Department of Health and Human Services, 1982.

CHAPTER 2. EPIDEMIC

1. A. Ochsner, The development of pulmonary surgery. *American Journal of Surgery* 1978; 135: 732–746.
2. M. E. DeBakey, In Memoriam: Dr. Ochsner the surgeon. *Journal of Thoracic and Cardiovascular Surgery* 1982; 84: 4–5.

CHAPTER 3. ENUMERATION

1. R. Doll and R. Peto, Mortality in relation to smoking: 20 years' observation on male British doctors. *British Medical Journal* 1976; 2: 1525–1536.
2. E. C. Hammond, Smoking in relation to mortality and morbidity: Findings in first thirty-four months of follow-up in a prospective study started in 1959. *Journal of the National Cancer Institute* 1964; 32: 1161–1188.
3. E. C. Hammond and D. Horn, Smoking and death rates: Report on 44

months of follow-up of 187,783 men. II. Death rates by cause. *Journal of the American Medical Association* 1958; 166: 1294–1308.

4. L. Garfinkel, O. Auerbach, and L. Joubert, Involuntary smoking and lung cancer: A case-control study. *Journal of the National Cancer Institute* 1985; 75: 463–469.

5. C. G. Humble et al., Marriage to a smoker and lung cancer risk. *American Journal of Public Health* 1987; 77: 598–602.

6. N. L. Benowitz, S. M. Hall et al., Smokers of low-yield cigarettes do not consume less nicotine. *New England Journal of Medicine* 1983; 309: 139–142.

7. D. W. Kaufman, S. P. Helmrich et al., Nicotine and carbon monoxide content of cigarette smoke and the risk of myocardial infarction in young men. *New England Journal of Medicine* 1983; 308: 409–413.

8. Church of Jesus Christ of Latter-Day Saints, *Doctrine and Covenants*. Salt Lake City, 1957 (Section 89).

9. J. L. Lyon et al., Cancer incidence in Mormons and non-Mormons in Utah during 1967–75. *Journal of the National Cancer Institute* 1980; 65: 1055–1061.

10. J. E. Enstrom, Cancer mortality among California Mormons, 1968–1975. *Journal of the National Cancer Institute* 1980; 65: 1073–1082.

11. E. Lorenz, Radioactivity and lung cancer: Critical review of lung cancer in miners of Schneeberg and Joachimsthal. *Journal of the National Cancer Institute* 1944; 5: 1–15.

12. G. Saccomanno, V. Archer et al., Histologic types of lung cancer among uranium miners. *Cancer* 1971; 27: 515–523. J. M. Samet, D. M. Kutvirt, et al., Uranium mining and lung cancer in Navajo men. *New England Journal of Medicine* 1984; 310: 1481–1484.

13. E. P. Radford and K. G. St. Clair, Lung cancer in Swedish iron miners exposed to low doses of radon daughters. *New England Journal of Medicine* 1984; 310: 1485–1494.

14. J. Horacek, Der Joachimstaler Lungenkrebs nach dem zweiten Weltkrieg (The lung cancer of Joachimsthal since the Second World War). *Zeitschrift für Krebsforschung* (*Journal for Cancer Research*) 1969; 72: 52–56.

15. M. Goldsmith, How serious is the indoor radiation hazard? *Journal of the American Medical Association* 1985; 258: 578–579. (Also): Council on Scientific Affairs. Radon in homes. ibid., 668–672; N. H. Harley, Radon and lung cancer in mines and homes. *New England Journal of Medicine* 1984; 310: 1525–1526.

16. E. Silverberg and J. Lubera. Cancer statistics, 1989. *CA-A Cancer Journal for Clinicians* 1989; 39: 3–20.

17. I. J. Selikoff and E. C. Hammond. Asbestos-associated disease in United States shipyards. *CA-A Cancer Journal for Clinicians* 1978; 28: 87.

18. Silverberg and Lubera, Cancer Statistics.

19. A.R. Al-Awadi and H. A. Al-Mumen. Progress against smoking in Kuwait. *New York State Journal of Medicine* 1985; 85: 466–467; D.C. Sokal. Cigarette advertising in the Third World. *New York State Journal of Medicine* 1985; 85: 467–468.

20. Ibid.; J. Madeley, How smoking promotes hunger. *New York State Journal of Medicine* 1985; 85: 442–443.

21. P. Schmeisser, Pushing Cigarettes Overseas. *New York Times Magazine* (July 10, 1988): 18.

22. T-C. Wu et al., Pulmonary hazards of smoking marijuana as compared with tobacco. *New England Journal of Medicine* 1988; 318: 347–351.

23. M. Markman et al., Association between HLA-Bw44 and small-cell carcinoma of the lung. *New England Journal of Medicine* 1982; 307: 1087.

24. J. Cairns, *Cancer: Science and Society*. San Francisco, W. H. Freeman and Company, 1978, 173.

25. M. S. Menkes et al., Serum beta-carotene, vitamins A and E, selenium, and the risk of lung cancer. *New England Journal of Medicine* 1986; 315: 1250–1254.

26. W. C. Willett et al., Relation of serum vitamins A and E and carotenoids to the risk of cancer. *New England Journal of Medicine* 1984; 310: 430–434.

CHAPTER 4. SOME YOUNG PATIENTS

1. E. J. Cassell, The nature of suffering and the goals of medicine. *New England Journal of Medicine* 1982; 306: 639–645.

CHAPTER 5. YOUTH IS DIFFERENT

1. R. W. Miller and F. W. McKay, Decline in US childhood cancer mortality, 1950 through 1980. *Journal of the American Medical Association* 1984; 251: 1567–1570.

2. G. E. Hartman and S. J. Shochat, Primary pulmonary neoplasms of childhood: A review. *Annals of Thoracic Surgery* 1983; 36: 108–119.

3. A. Kennedy, Lung cancer in young adults. *British Journal of Diseases of the Chest* 1972; 66: 147–154; J. S. Putnam. Lung cancer in young adults. *Journal of the American Medical Association* 1977; 238: 35–36; L. DeCaro and J. R. Benfield, Lung cancer in young persons. *Journal of Thoracic and Cardiovascular Surgery* 1982; 83: 372–376; J. H. Pemberton, D. M. Nagorney, J. C. Gilmore, et al., Bronchogenic carcinoma in patients younger than 40 years. *Annals of Thoracic Surgery* 1983; 36: 509–515; A. J. Larrieu, W. R. E. Jamieson, et al., Carcinoma of the lung in patients under 40 years of age. *American Journal of Surgery* 1985; 149: 602–605.

4. M. Kyriakos and B. Webber, Cancer of the lung in young men. *Journal of Thoracic and Cardiovascular Surgery* 1974; 67: 634–648.

5. See note 3.
6. Pemberton et al., Bronchogenic carcinoma.
7. Larrieu et al., Carcinoma of the lung.
8. S. M. Teeter, F. F. Holmes et al., Lung carcinoma in the elderly population: Influence of histology on the inverse relationship of stage to age. *Cancer* 1987; 60: 1331–1336.

CHAPTER 6. NATURAL HISTORY OF THE DISEASE
1. R. G. Vincent et al., The changing histopathology of lung cancer: A review of 1682 cases. *Cancer* 1977; 39: 1647–1655.

CHAPTER 7. WHY ME?
1. C. P. Snow, *The Two Cultures: And A Second Look*. Cambridge and New York: Cambridge University Press, 1963, p. 72.
2. H. Simon, Cobalt Blue. *New England Journal of Medicine* 1986; 314: 587.

CHAPTER 8. DIAGNOSIS
1. American Cancer Society, Guidelines for the cancer-related checkup: Recommendations and rationale. *CA: A Cancer Journal for Clinicians* 1980; 30: 199–207.
2. M. H. Melamed et al., Impact of early detection on the clinical course of lung cancer. *Surgical Clinics of North America* 1987; 67: 909–924.

CHAPTER 10. SECONDARY TREATMENT
1. M. H. Cohen et al., Is immediate radiation therapy indicated for patients with unresectable non-small cell lung cancer? No. *Cancer Treatment Reports* 1983; 67: 333–336; J. D. Cox et al., Is immediate chest radiotherapy obligatory for any or all patients with unresectable non-small cell carcinoma of the lung? Yes. *Cancer Treatment Reports* 1983; 67: 327–331.
2. (Collaborative Study), Preoperative irradiation of cancer of the lung: Final report of a therapeutic trial. *Cancer* 1975; 36: 914–925.
3. H. E. Skipper et al., Experimental evaluation of potential anticancer agents. XIII. On the criteria and kinetics associated with "curability" of experimental leukemia. *Cancer Chemotherapy Reports* 1964; 35: 1–111.
4. R. K. Oye and M. F. Shapiro, Reporting results from chemotherapy trials: Does response make a difference in patient survival? *Journal of the American Medical Association* 1984; 252: 2722–2725.
5. E. Rapp et al., Chemotherapy can prolong survival in patients with advanced non-small-cell lung cancer: Report of a Canadian multicenter randomized trial. *Journal of Clinical Oncology* 1988; 6: 633–641.

CHAPTER 12. SEVERAL SUCCESSFUL CASES

1. G. A. Patterson et al., Significance of metastatic disease in subaortic lymph nodes. *Annals of Thoracic Surgery* 1987; 43: 155–159.

2. D. J. Magilligan, Jr., et al., Surgical approach to lung cancer with solitary cerebral metastasis: Twenty-five years' experience. *Annals of Thoracic Surgery* 1986; 42: 360–364.

3. L. G. Rigler. A roentgen study of the evolution of carcinoma of the lung. *Journal of Thoracic Surgery* 1957; 34: 283–297.

CHAPTER 13. FACTORS OF CURABILITY

1. D. E. Williams et al., Survival of patients surgically treated for stage I lung cancer. *Journal of Thoracic and Cardiovascular Surgery* 1981; 82: 70–76; N. Martini, E. J. Beattie, Results of surgical treatment of stage I lung cancer. *Journal of Thoracic and Cardiovascular Surgery* 1977; 74: 499–505.

2. J. D. Steele et al., Survival in males with bronchogenic carcinomas resected as asymptomatic solitary pulmonary nodules. *Annals of Thoracic Surgery* 1966; 2: 368–376; R. J. Jackman et al., Survival rates in peripheral bronchogenic carcinomas up to four centimeters in diameter presenting as solitary pulmonary nodules. *Journal of Thoracic and Cardiovascular Surgery* 1969; 57: 1–8.

3. O. C. Simonton et al., *Getting Well Again*: A step-by-step, self-help guide to overcoming cancer for patients and their families. Los Angeles: J. P. Tarcher, 1978.

4. R. M. Mack. Lessons from living with cancer. *New England Journal of Medicine* 1984; 311: 1640–1644.

5. Obituaries, *Journal of the American Medical Association* 1986; 255: 2687.

6. B. R. Cassileth et al., Psychosocial correlates of survival in adult malignant disease? *New England Journal of Medicine* 1985; 312: 1551–1555.

7. M. Angell, Disease as a reflection of the psyche. *New England Journal of Medicine* 1985; 312: 1570–1572.

8. T. C. Everson and W. H. Cole. Spontaneous regression of cancer: Preliminary report. *Annals of Surgery* 1956; 144: 366–383.

9. J. W. Bell et al., Spontaneous regression of bronchogenic carcinoma with five year survival. *Journal of Thoracic and Cardiovascular Surgery* 1964; 48: 984–990.

10. J. E. Jesseph, M. D. Personal communication, 1977.

11. Everson and Cole, Spontaneous regression of cancer; Bell et al., Spontaneous regression.

CHAPTER 14. THE VARIANT: SMALL-CELL CARCINOMA

1. W. Fox and J. G. Scadding. Medical Research Council comparative trial of

surgery and radiotherapy for primary treatment of small-celled or oat-celled carcinoma of the bronchus: Ten year follow-up. *Lancet* 1973; 2: 63–65.

2. R. T. Eagan et al., Combination chemotherapy and radiation therapy in small cell carcinoma. *Cancer* 1973; 32: 371–379.

3. A. Johnston-Early et al., Smoking abstinence and small cell lung cancer survival: An association. *Journal of the American Medical Association* 1980; 244: 2175–2179.

4. S. Davis et al., Long-term survival in small cell carcinoma of the lung: A population experience. *Journal of Clinical Oncology* 1985; 3: 80–91; C. F. Mountain, Operation for small-cell carcinoma revisited. *Journal of Clinical Oncology* 1987; 5: 687–688.

5. J. A. Meyer, Five year survival in treated Stage I and II small cell carcinoma of the lung. *Annals of Thoracic Surgery* 1986; 42: 668–669.

CHAPTER 15. REASONABLE THERAPEUTIC INTENSITY

1. W. L. Shirer, *The Rise and Fall of the Third Reich*. New York, Simon and Schuster, 1960, pp. 979 ff.

2. Nuremberg Tribunal, *Trials of War Criminals Before the Nuremberg Military Tribunals Under Control Council Law*. Number 10, Volume 2. Washington, D. C., U.S. Government Printing Office, 1949, p. 181.

3. World Medical Association, Recommendations guiding medical doctors in biomedical research involving human subjects. Declaration adopted by the 18th World Medical Assembly, Helsinki, 1964; Revised by the 29th W. M. A., Tokyo, 1975. (Known as the "Declaration of Helsinki").

4. Preliminary Report: Findings from the aspirin component of the ongoing physicians' health study. *New England Journal of Medicine* 1988; 318: 262–264.

5. S. Davis et al., Participants in prospective, randomized clinical trials for resected non-small-cell lung cancer have improved survival compared with nonparticipants in such trials. *Cancer* 1985; 56: 1710–1718.

6. R. E. Johnson et al., "Total" therapy for small cell carcinoma of the lung. *Annals of Thoracic Surgery* 1978; 25: 510–515.

7. W. J. Mackillop et al., The use of expert surrogates to evaluate clinical trials in non-small-cell lung cancer. *British Journal of Cancer* 1986; 54: 661–667.

8. H. H. Hansen, Advanced non-small-cell lung cancer: To treat or not to treat? *Journal of Clinical Oncology* 1987; 5: 1711–1712.

CHAPTER 16. PRODUCT LIABILITY

1. R. A. Daynard, Tobacco liability legislation as a cancer control strategy. *Journal of the National Cancer Institute* 1988; 80: 9–13.

2. M. Z. Edell and S. M. Gisser, Cipollone v. Liggett Group, Inc.: The applica-

tion of theories of liability in current cigarette litigation. *N.Y. State Journal of Medicine* 1985; 85: 318–321.
3. New York Times News Service, June 2, 1988.
4. A Bum Rap For The Tobacco Companies, Universal Press Syndicate, June 1988.
5. The aphorism, "War is too important to be left to the generals," has been attributed variously to Charles-Maurice de Talleyrand (1754–1838), Aristide Briand (1862–1932), and Georges Clemenceau (1841–1929). At least it seems to have been uttered by a Frenchman.

CHAPTER 17. ADDICTION

1. N. L. Benowitz. Pharmacologic aspects of cigarette smoking and nicotine addiction. *New England Journal of Medicine* 1988; 319: 1318–1329.
2. Ibid.
3. R. C. S. Trahair, Giving up cigarettes: 222 case studies. *Medical Journal of Australia* 1967; 1: 929–932.
4. *The Health Consequences of Smoking: Nicotine Addiction.* A Report of the Surgeon General. Washington, D. C., Department of Health and Human Services, 1988.
5. World Health Organization, *5th Review of Psychoactive Substances for International Control.* Geneva, World Health Organization, 1981.
6. American Psychiatric Association, *Diagnostic and Statistical Manual of Mental Disorders*, Third Edition (DSM-III). Washington, D. C., American Psychiatric Association, 1987.
7. Trahair, Giving up cigarettes.
8. *The Health Consequences of Smoking.*
9. T. E. Kottke et al., Attributes of successful smoking cessation interventions in medical practice: A meta-analysis of 39 controlled trials. *Journal of American Medical Association* 1988; 259: 2883–2889.
10. Trahair, Giving up cigarettes.
11. J. D. Killen et al., Are heavy smokers different from light smokers? *Journal of American Medical Association* 1988; 260: 1581–1585.
12. L. T. Kozlowski et al., Comparing tobacco cigarette dependence with other drug dependencies. *Journal of American Medical Association* 1989; 261: 898–901.
13. M. T. Southgate, Making love with Death. *Journal of American Medical Association* 1986; 255: 1054.
14. Ibid.

CHAPTER 18. UNORTHODOX OR "ALTERNATIVE" TREATMENTS

1. H. M. Hoxsey, *You Don't Have To Die.* New York: Milestone Books, 1956.

2. Editorial: Gerson's cancer treatment. *Journal of the American Medical Association* 1946; 132: 645–646.
3. Editorial: Cancer and the need for facts. (*Ibid.*) 1949; 139: 93–98.
4. J. F. Holland, The Krebiozen story: Is cancer quackery dead? *Journal of American Medical Association* 1967; 200: 213–218.
5. C. G. Moertel and others. A clinical trial of amygdalin (Laetrile) in the treatment of cancer. *New England Journal of Medicine* 1982; 306: 201–206.
6. American Cancer Society. *Unproven Methods of Cancer Management.* New York: American Cancer Society, 1982.
7. Moertel et al., Clinical trial.
8. N. M. Ellison a et al., Special report on Laetrile: Results of the National Cancer Institute's retrospective Laetrile analysis. *New England Journal of Medicine* 1978; 299: 549–552.
9. Moertel et al., Clinical trial.
10. Diagnostic and Therapeutic Technology Assessment: Immunoaugmentative Therapy. *Journal of American Medical Association* 1988 ; 259: 3477–78. S. L. Nightingale, Immunoaugmentative Therapy: Assessing an untested therapy (Editorial). (*Ibid.*) 259: 3457–58.
11. Diagnostic and Therapeutic Technology Assessment.

CHAPTER 19. ECONOMICS, GOVERNMENT, AND THE MEDIA
1. L. Fritschler, *Smoking and Politics.* New York: Appleton-Century-Crofts, 1975.
2. J. Cairns, The treatment of diseases and the war against cancer. *Scientific American* 1985; 253: 51–59.
3. P. Schmeisser, Pushing cigarettes overseas. *New York Times Magazine,* July 10, 1988, p. 16 ff.
4. J. Cairns. The treatment of diseases and the war against cancer.
5. A. Bailey, The epidemiology of bronchial carcinoma. In M. Bates, FRCS., *Bronchial Carcinoma: An Integrated Approach to Diagnosis and Management.* Berlin, New York, and Tokyo: Springer-Verlag, 1984.
6. A. Mangiacasale, Whig-Standard will refuse ads for tobacco products. *The Whig-Standard* (Kingston), November 27, 1984.
7. No tobacco promotion. *The Globe and Mail* (Toronto), August 27, 1986.
8. G. Gitlitz, Cigarette advertising and *The New York Times:* An ethical issue that's not fit to print? *New York State Journal of Medicine* 1983; 83: 1284–1291.
9. C. S. Kitchens, Cigarette ads in the *Ladies' Home Journal. New England Journal of Medicine* 1984; 311: 51–52.
10. J. J. O'Connor, Women top cig target. *Advertising Age* 1981; 52: #9; 93.
11. A. Sobczynski, Marketers clamor to offer lady a cigarette. *Advertising Age,* January 31, 1983, pp M 14–16.

12. "You've Come A Long Way, Baby!" *Philip Morris Magazine,* Winter 1985.
13. E. M. Whelan et al., Analysis of coverage of tobacco hazards in women's magazines. *Journal of Public Health Policy* 1981; 2: 28–35.
14. *Consumers' Reports.* September 1987.
15. K. E. Warner. Cigarette advertising and media coverage of smoking and health. (Special Report). *New England Journal of Medicine* 1985; 312: 384–388.
16. Common Cause. News letter to membership, June 1988.
17. *Washington Post,* April 7, 1988: pp. E1, E4.
18. The business of smoking. *New York State Journal of Medicine* 1983; 83: 1324–1332.
19. A. Chesterfield-Evans, BUGA-UP (Billboard-Utilizing Graffitists Against Unhealthy Promotions): An Australian movement to end cigarette advertising. *New York State Journal of Medicine* 1983; 83: 1333–1334.

CHAPTER 20. PROSPECTS FOR THE FUTURE

1. I. H. Krakoff, Cancer chemotherapeutic agents. *CA, A Cancer Journal for Clinicians* 1987; 37: 93–105.
2. H. B. Hewitt et al., A critique of the evidence for active host defence against cancer, based on personal studies of 27 murine tumors of spontaneous origin. *British Journal of Cancer* 1976; 33: 241–250. D. W. Weiss, Animal models of cancer immunotherapy: Questions of relevance. *Cancer Treatment Reports* 1980; 64: 481–485.
3. R. T. Prehn, Relationship of tumor immunogenicity to concentration of the inducing oncogen. *Journal of the National Cancer Institute* 1975; 55: 189–190.
4. R. B. Herberman and H. T. Holden, Natural cell-mediated immunity. *Advances in Cancer Research* 1978; 27: 305–377.
5. D. A. Morgan et al., Selective in vitro growth of T lymphocytes from normal human bone marrow. *Science* 1976; 193: 1007–1008.
6. S. A. Rosenberg et al., Observations on the systemic administration of autologous lymphokine-activated killer cells and recombinant interleukin-2 to patients with metastatic cancer. *New England Journal of Medicine* 1985; 313: 1485–1492. S. A. Rosenberg et al., A new approach to the adoptive immunotherapy of cancer with tumor-infiltrating lymphocytes. *Science* 1986; 233: 1318–1321.

APPENDIX A. DOUBLING TIME AS A MEASURE OF TUMOR GROWTH RATE

1. V. P. Collins et al., Observations on growth rates of human tumors. *American Journal of Roentgenology* 1956; 76: 988–1000.
2. Ibid.
3. M. Schwartz, A biomathematical approach to clinical tumor growth. *Cancer* 1961; 14: 1272–1294.

4. D. M. Geddes, The natural history of lung cancer: A review based on rates of tumor growth. *British Journal of Diseases of the Chest* 1979; 73: 1–17; T. Mizuno et al., Comparison of actual survivorship after treatment with survivorship predicted by actual tumor-volume doubling time from tumor volume at first observation. *Cancer* 1984 ; 53: 2716–2720.

5. A. K. Laird, Dynamics of tumor growth. *British Journal of Cancer* 1964; 18: 490–502.

6. J. A. Meyer, Growth rate versus prognosis in resected primary bronchogenic carcinomas. *Cancer* 1973; 31: 1468–1472.

7. W. L. Joseph, D. L. Morton, and P. C. Adkins, Prognostic significance of doubling time in evaluating operability in pulmonary metastatic disease. *Journal of Thoracic and Cardiovascular Surgery* 1971; 61: 23–32.

APPENDIX B. HISTOLOGIC TYPES

1. World Health Organization: The World Health Organization histological typing of lung tumors. *American Journal of Clinical Pathology* 1982; 77: 123–136.

2. R. G. Vincent et al., The changing histopathology of lung cancer: A review of 1682 cases. *Cancer* 1977; 39: 1647–1655.

3. E. S. Wright and C. M. Couves, Radiation-induced carcinoma of the lung: the St. Lawrence tragedy. *Journal of Thoracic and Cardiovascular Surgery* 1977; 74: 495–498.

4. Vincent et al., Changing histopathology.

Glossary

acid-fast adj. (Applied to organisms, or bacilli.) A group of bacilli, principally the organism causing tuberculosis, and related species. The distinguishing feature is that they take up a red stain (fuchsin) and retain it through subsequent acid washing; hence the staining is acid-resistant or acid-fast. Other organisms and tissues do not hold the stain through acid washing; as a result the acid-fast organisms stand out in bright red color during microscopic examination of stained smears.

'ad-e-no-'car-ci-'no-ma n. (See also *carcinoma*.) A carcinoma that arises from gland tissue and preserves some of the distinctive structural pattern of glands in microscopic section. Adenocarcinomas may arise in breast tissue, prostate, in the lining of the gastrointestinal tract as in stomach or colon; other glandular structures such as thyroid, ovaries, pancreas; and in mucous glands lining the bronchial tubes of the lungs. In this volume, unless otherwise noted, the word refers to primary adenocarcinoma of the lung, one of the cell types of lung cancer.

ad-'he-sions plural n. (Seldom used in the singular.) State of abnormal sticking together of tissue surfaces, by multiple sites of fibrous union, usually as the result of an old inflammatory process. Adhesions often form between the peritoneal surfaces in the abdomen, the pleural surfaces in the chest, and so on.

'ad-ju-vant adj. (From Latin, "to aid.") In cancer treatment, a second mode of therapy given following the primary treatment; as, adjuvant chemotherapy may be given following surgery in certain cases of breast cancer.

ad-'ren-al glands n. (From Latin, "adjacent to the kidney.") Paired (left and right) glands in the upper abdomen, one lying just above each kidney; they secrete adrenaline or epinephrine as well as other hormones; fairly frequent sites of metastasis from cancer of the lung.

'al-ka-loid n. Any of numerous compounds derived from plants, chemically basic in pure form, usually with powerful physiologic effects on the body; examples are the naturally occurring narcotics morphine, codeine, cannabinol; also vincristine and vinblastine used in cancer chemotherapy.

'al-lo-ge-'ne-ic adj. (From Greek, "having other genes.") Applied to individuals

**In this glossary the syllable accent is noted by the mark ' preceding the syllable.

of the same species, not closely related, and sufficiently different genetically so that they would reject each other's tissues after grafting; the normal state between human beings with the exception of identical twins, while parent-child and sibling-sibling genetic matches may sometimes be closer than simple allogeneic matches. (See also *syngeneic*.)

'al-lo-graft n. A tissue or organ graft between unrelated individuals of the same species, not accepted by the new host except after suppression of the immune response.

an- aer-'ob-ic gly-'col-y-sis adj. and n. Name for the biochemical pathway by which the basic sugar (glucose) can be partially broken down in the absence of oxygen (anaerobically), yielding the host a small amount of energy. The pathway ends with lactic acid, which accumulates with detrimental effect until or unless oxygen becomes available to allow the reactions to proceed to water and carbon dioxide; this aerobic chemical pathway is productive of much larger amounts of energy.

an-a-'plas-tic adj., generally applied to carcinomas, or to tumors more generally. (The term is more or less synonymous with "undifferentiated.") A malignant tumor showing a generally disordered, even chaotic, cellular structure on microscopic examination; not fitting the structural pattern of better "differentiated" tumor types. Anaplastic tumors tend to be more malignant in their behavior.

'ant-acids n. Alkaline or basic medications taken by mouth to neutralize stomach acids, as for relief of ulcer pain, "heartburn" resulting from a hiatus hernia, and the like.

'an-ti-bod-y n. A protein of the globulin class, manufactured by the immune system as the unique and specific neutralizer of an antigen to which the host has been sensitized.

'an-ti-gen n. A compound, usually a protein but sometimes a carbohydrate or other, recognized as foreign to the body, and as a result able to provoke an immune reaction and the production of antibodies.

an-ti-'sep-sis n. In surgery, the system of disinfection of surgeons' hands, the patient's skin, all instruments and drapes with phenol (carbolic acid) as developed by Joseph Lister (1877), professor of surgery at King's College Hospital, London, later raised to the peerage as Baron Lister. Antiseptic surgery began to point the way toward control of infection in surgical wounds; superseded by aseptic surgery.

a-'ort-a n. The great artery leaving the left ventricle of the heart, carrying oxygenated blood to the entire body.

a-'sep-sis n. In surgery, the extension and refinement of antisepsis; the concept of making and preserving a sterile field for the operation, rather than attempting to cleanse a field by spraying it with phenol. In practice, it means that all drapes and instruments have been sterilized by steam (autoclaving), the surgeons' hands and the patient's skin have been thoroughly scrubbed, and the surgeons wear sterile gloves.

a-'symp-tom-'at-ic adj. Not experiencing any symptoms (if applied to a patient); or not causing any symptoms (if applied to a tumor or disease process).

at-el-'ec-ta-sis n. Loose meaning is collapse or partial collapse of a lung; but more properly, the word implies airless collapse, resulting from obstruction of the bronchus to that area of lung. The lung involved by atelectasis shows increased opacity on X-ray examination, and marked loss of volume.

'at-ri-um n. (From Latin, the entrance hall of a house.) One of the two (left and right) upper chambers of the mammalian heart; veins from the body return blood into the right atrium, which in turn empties into the right ventricle and thence to the pulmonary artery; while the pulmonary veins return oxygenated blood from the lungs into the left atrium which drains into the left ventricle and thence to the aorta, the great artery to the body. Atrium is not precisely synonymous with auricle although the latter word often is misused for it.

a-'typ-i-cal adj. Not normal, abnormal; in cytology and microscopic examination of tissues generally, applied to cells that show changes in the direction of malignancy, but are not yet clearly malignant.

'bi-op-sy n. (From Greek, "to see, examine from life," as opposed to necropsy, "examine from death.") 1. A small portion of tissue removed from a suspicious-appearing lesion or organ for microscopic examination, principally for the diagnosis of malignancy. 2. The procedure of obtaining a biopsy specimen.

bone scan n. Image of the skeletal system made following intravenous injection of a tiny (tracer) dose of a radioactive element, technetium 99, which is quickly taken up in the bones; used primarily to examine for possible tumor involvement of the bones.

'bron-chi-al ad-e-'no-mas adj. and n. (Compare with the two following definitions.) A small group of tumors arising from the bronchi, generally of low grade malignancy and for the most part curable. They bear no relation to smoking or radon inhalation. Should not be classified as lung cancer because their behavior and prognosis are generally different.

'bron-cho-'gen-ic 'car-ci-'no-ma adj. and n. Carcinoma (q.v.) arising from the epithelial lining of the bronchus; the phrase is generally synonymous with lung cancer since the cancers actually arise from the bronchi.

'bron-chus n. (plural *bronchi*; diminutive *bronchiole*, a small bronchus). Tubular passageway through which air passes into and out of the lungs. The two main bronchi (one leading to each lung) are formed by the division of the trachea, or windpipe, which is single and located in the midline of the neck and chest. In successive branchings, the main bronchi give off lobar bronchi, then segmental, then smaller and smaller branches in the manner of branches of a tree.

'bron-cho-scope n. A slim, lighted optical instrument designed for examination of the interior of the bronchial "tree," as far out as the orifices of the segmental bronchi. Biopsies may be taken through the scope of any abnormal tissue visualized within the bronchial passageway. Older models are in the form of a rigid tube; but newer designs are slim and flexible, using the principles of fiber-optic images and lighting.

'bron-'chos-co-py n. The procedure, of examination of the interior of the bronchi, by means of a bronchoscope.

'cal-ci-fi-'ca-tion n. The process of deposition of insoluble salts of calcium, principally calcium carbonate and calcium phosphates, in tissues within the body. Bones are calcified already, but deposition may occur in other tissues, often after chronic infection or other gradually destructive processes. Calcification usually is visible in X-ray films as a density much greater than that of soft tissues.

'can-cer n. Popular inclusive term for all malignant tumors (See also *tumors.*) For precise meaning, medical terminology distinguishes between carcinomas, sarcomas, lymphomas, and also between their individual types.

'car-ci-'no-ma n. A malignant tumor (hence, in popular terms, a cancer), which arises originally from epithelial or surface-lining cells, such as those of the skin, the lining membranes of the stomach or intestinal tract, the lining of the bronchial tubes in the lung, the lining of pocket-like structures of glands, and the like. Behavior differs in certain ways from that of malignancies arising from other tissues (See also *sarcoma.*)

'car-ci-no-'gen-ic adj. Able to cause cancer in a living organism; a property of certain chemicals, certain virus infections, solar or nuclear radiation.

ca-'rot-e-noids plural n. (See also *retinoids.*) Biochemical precursors of vitamin A, being investigated for possible cancer-preventive effects.

'cat-gut n. Cords or strings prepared from the smooth-muscle layer of animal intestine, usually of sheep; cats were never used for this preparation and the origin of the term is obscure; used for violin strings, tennis rackets, and so on, but in surgery used for sutures and ligatures. The advantage was that being animal tissue, the strands would eventually be absorbed within the body (absorbable suture, in contrast to cotton, silk, nylon, and other materials that are nonabsorbable.) Catgut has been largely replaced by synthetic absorbable suture which is stronger, more uniform.

cell type n. Identifies individual varieties of cancer of a given organ, on the basis of the cells making up the tumor. "Lung cancer," for example, is not a single type, but includes adenocarcinoma of the lung, squamous-cell carcinoma, large-cell and small-cell undifferentiated carcinomas, plus other less common types.

chest n. That portion of the body contained within the rib cage; upper boundary at the level of the first ribs, approximately at level of the collar-bones; lower boundary the thin muscular sheet called the diaphragm, separating chest cavity from abdominal cavity. The chest contains primarily the centers of respiration (lungs) and circulation (heart and great vessels), intimately involved with each other.

chest wall n. The "cage" formed by the ribs for protection of the heart and lungs, plus both thin and heavy muscle layers attached to the ribs.

'chrom-o-some n. A structure in the nucleus of living cells, plant or animal, containing a long spiral double strand of deoxyribonucleic acid (DNA), the compound that codes and transmits genetic information. Prior to cell division, the strands separate and each replicates its mirror-image strand, forming a full complement of chromosomes for each of the two resulting cells. Normal resting human somatic (body) cells contain forty-six chromosomes, in twenty-three pairs, including the two designated XX and XY which determine the sex of the organism.

colo-'rect-al carcinoma adj. and n. Carcinoma (adenocarcinoma in type) arising in the colon or rectum, that is, in the large intestine. Second leading cause of cancer death among men in the United States (after lung cancer), and third among women (after lung and breast cancer).

computerized to-mo-'graph-ic (CT) scan adjs. and n. Relatively new method of body imaging, in which many transverse X-ray beams are synthesized by computer to produce a series of images, each depicting a cross section of the body, ordinarily 1 cm apart. Examined in sequence, these can give an unusually complete picture of the internal organs.

cy-'tol-o-gy n. Properly, the study of cells: their biology, metabolism, growth, and death. In clinical medicine, the microscopic examination of isolated cells, mainly with the objective of identifying malignant cells when present; more properly, cytologic examination, as of Papanicolaou smears from the uterine cervix, or from sputum.

'di-a-phragm n. (The letter "g" is silent.) A thin sheet of muscle and flat tendon, which separates the chest cavity from the abdominal cavity; an essential muscle in the breathing mechanism, hence also in coughing, speech, and much else.

dis-'sem-in-a-tion n. The spreading of cancer cells away from the site of origin, which cells later can grow into metastases; in particular, distant spread via the blood stream.

'dis-tal adj. Farther away from the center (of the body), as opposed to *proximal*, closer to the center. The hand is at the distal end of the arm, the shoulder at the proximal.

em-phy-'se-ma n. A disease process producing progressive degenerative changes in the lung, with resultant increasing shortness of breath, pulmonary insufficiency, plus enlargement and stiffening of the chest, called the "barrel chest" configuration. Precipitated largely by smoking, although an individual biochemical predisposition has been identified.

em-py-'e-ma n. (From Latin, "containing pus"; properly, empyema thoracis, "pus contained within the chest.") Infection with accumulation of pus within the pleural space; may occur as a complication of pneumonia, penetrating wounds of the chest, or following surgery on the lung; serious complication when following surgery; generally demands surgical drainage and placement of a drainage tube.

en-do-'me-tri-'o-sis n. Presence of scattered implants of endometrium, the distinctive mucous membrane lining the uterus, elsewhere in the abdomen, generally on the surfaces of the intestine, bladder, or abdominal wall; also, a syndrome of various and often vague abdominal symptoms resulting from such implantation.

ep-i-'dur-al space adj. and n. Thin buffer space lying just outside the dura mater, a tough protective membrane which envelops the brain and spinal cord. Nerves leaving the brain or cord for the body pass out through the epidural space; the nerves may be temporarily blocked here by injection of local anesthetic solutions into the space.

ep-i-'the-li-um n. (Adj., epithelial). Thin lining layer of a body surface, internal or external, made up of uniform cells generally having a continuous high rate of replacement; examples are the epidermis or outer layer of the skin, and membranes lining the interior of the mouth, the intestinal tract, or the bronchial tubes of the lung. The interior secreting surface of glands also is made up of epithelium. *Carcinomas* arise from epithelial cells, in contrast to *sarcomas* which arise from cells of other tissues.

er-y-'sip-e-las n. (From Greek and Latin, "red skin.") A spreading infection of the tissues under the skin by a strain of Streptococcus, accompanied by high fever and profound malaise; practically unknown since the advent of penicillin.

'fe-brile adj. Feverish.

fellow n. In this context, a young physician taking advanced specialty training; fellows in cardiology, oncology, and so on, may be taking additional training over and above their residency training in internal medicine; also, trainees in cardiac and thoracic surgery often are designated fellows, beyond their residency training in surgery.

'flu-or-o-scope n. An X-ray apparatus constructed so that the image formed by X-ray beams may be watched on a screen, resembling a television screen in the more modern types.

frozen section n. Method of quick-freezing tissue from a biopsy and cutting fine, almost invisibly thin sections which are fixed on a glass slide and stained for microscopic examination; useful when the diagnosis of malignancy must be confirmed or eliminated during an operation, as a guide to what needs to be done.

general anesthesia adj. and n. Anesthesia which maintains the patient in an unconscious state ("asleep"); as opposed to local anesthesia, "freezing" of an area of skin by injection of appropriate agents (such as novocain) while the subject remains awake.

'gen-o-type n. The identity and specific arrangement of genes within the chromosomes, which determine the behavior and characteristics of a cell, for example a cancer cell.

gross adj. (adv., *grossly*). Attributes or characteristics of an organ or a tumor as seen by the unaided eye, or as palpated by the hand; as opposed to characteristics as seen through the microscope. A tumor is examined *grossly* by the surgeon, both *grossly* and microscopically by the pathologist.

he-'mop-ty-sis n. (From Greek, "spitting blood.") The meaning is different in English medical terminology; the word implies coughing up of blood, not just spitting.

'hep-a-'ti-tis n. Any one of several virus infections causing damage to the liver, usually with fever, jaundice, weakness and malaise; hepatitis B is transmitted through blood or blood products, needle sticks, and the like, and results in long-term damage to the liver and the risk of liver cancer.

hi-'at-us hernia n. *Hernia* signifies protrusion of internal organs outside a body cavity, abdomen, chest, or other, through a defect in the wall of the cavity, although the protruded organ still remains within the body. *Hiatus hernia* signifies protrusion of the upper end of the stomach into the chest, through an opening in the diaphragm called the esophageal hiatus; the symptoms of hiatus hernia are chiefly those of heartburn and regurgitation.

'hi-lum n. The "root" of the lung; a cluster of structures which include, on each side, the main bronchus and the main pulmonary artery to that lung, two pulmonary veins draining each lung, plus some nerves and lesser structures.

'his-to-log-ic type See *cell type.*

'hy-per-ven-ti-la-tion n. Literally, "over-breathing"; deep, rapid, forceful breathing ordinarily a sign of overpowering agitation or tension; has the effect of severely reducing levels of carbon dioxide normally dissolved in the blood, which in turn may precipitate alarming symptoms seemingly not related to the agitation.

in-ter-'cos-tal nerve (s) adj. and n. (From Latin, "between the ribs.") Under each rib runs a nerve, which has left the spinal cord at the appropriate level, and transmits pain sensation from a comparable segment of the chest wall and skin. There are also intercostal muscle layers, arteries, and veins; all similarly located "between the ribs."

'is-o-ge-'ne-ic adj. (also, isologous). (From Greek, "having the same genes.") Applied to individuals so closely related as to have the same genetic pattern, as in human identical twins, and therefore able to freely accept tissue or organ grafts from each other (isografts). Not strictly synonymous with *syngeneic*, which refers to animal strains that are highly inbred, but in whom subtle or minor genetic differences might remain.

killer cell n. A specialized lymphocyte (one of the classes of white blood cells) with the ability to seek out and kill cancer cells or virus-infected cells under appropriate conditions; called NK or natural-killer cell when occurring spontaneously in the body, or LAK (lymphokine-activated killer) cell when stimulated by the activator IL-2.

large-cell carcinoma n. (More properly, large-cell undifferentiated carcinoma). Another of the major cell types of lung cancer; a more heterogeneous group than the others in terms of microscopic appearance and clinical behavior; but its behavior tends to be more malignant than that of squamous cell carcinoma and adenocarcinoma. Almost without exception, closely related to a history of heavy smoking.

'lar-ynx n. (Rhymes with fair inks. Adjective: laryngeal, having to do with the larynx.) The structure popularly known as the "voice box," containing the vocal cords which form the sounds of speech; visible externally as the "Adam's apple." All air and smoke inhaled or exhaled passes through the larynx.

'le-sion n. A point of abnormal change in an organ or tissue; in cancer diagnosis and treatment, generally signifies an abnormality suspected to be a focus of cancer, as: metastatic lesions in the brain, for example, or bones.

'lig-ate v.t. To tie securely, as to ligate a bleeding vessel during an operation; the thread or cord used in doing so is a ligature (n.)

lobe n. A division of the lung, separated from the other lobes by clefts called fissures. The left lung has two lobes (upper and lower); the right lung has three (upper, middle, and lower).

lo-'bec-tomy n. Surgical operation, of removal of a lobe. (See *pneumonectomy* in contrast.)

'lu-cent adj. (From Latin, glowing or light-giving.) In radiology, a feature of the shadows on an X-ray film; applied to an area that allows increased passage of the X-ray beams through otherwise dense structures, such as bone; meaning that the lucent area has diminished density. (Also, lucency [noun], or radiolucency.)

lymph node n. (Sometimes called lymph gland, especially in Great Britain.) Small structure, in effect a capsule filled with lymphocytes, the immunologically active blood cells. Tiny vessels carry tissue fluid (lymph) into the node and also drain away beyond it, returning lymph into the veins. The lymph nodes may be thought of as stations in the host's defense system. Carcinoma cells escaping from a tumor are likely to lodge in the lymph nodes, then grow there, forming secondary tumors or "lymph node metastases."

lym-'phom-a n. Malignant tumor arising from the lymphocytes, white blood cells responsible for immune reactions plus other functions; some examples include leukemias, Hodgkin's disease, non-Hodgkin's lymphomas. Lymphomas generally are not suited to definitive treatment by surgery, but respond to radiation therapy and chemotherapy.

'me-di-a-'sti-num n. May be thought of as an enclosed compartment in the midline of the chest, separating the right and left pleural cavities which contain the lungs. The mediastinum encloses the heart and great vessels, the trachea or windpipe, the esophagus or gullet, and the thymus gland; also the main lymph channel (thoracic duct) and lesser channels, many lymph nodes, several nerves, and so on.

'me-di-a-'sti-'nos-co-py n. Surgical procedure, of limited exploration of the upper mediastinum looking for tumor involvement of the lymph nodes draining the lung; biopsies may be taken of any that appear abnormal or suspicious. A "positive" biopsy (showing tumor involving the mediastinal nodes) generally signifies a poor prognosis; but there can be a few carefully defined exceptions to this rule.

'mel-a-'no-ma n. (From Greek, "black tumor.") A type of malignant tumor, usually arising in the skin, usually containing black pigment, melanin, although pigment may be absent in a few cases. Tends to be highly malignant in its behavior.

me-'tas-ta-sis n. (plural *metastases*.) A point of spread of carcinoma or sarcoma to another organ or site; spread may have occurred via the blood stream to a distant site (distant metastasis), or via lymphatic channels to regional lymph nodes (lymphatic metastasis). Distant metastasis generally signifies incurability, with hardly any exceptions; lymphatic metastasis has a severely adverse effect on prognosis but does not necessarily mean incurability.

mi-'tos-is n. (plural *mitoses*; adjective *mitotic*, having to do with mitosis.) The process by which a cell divides into two daughter cells, each containing the full complement of chromosomes. Mitosis takes place in four stages which are identifiable microscopically. Occurs in malignant as well as normal cells, but abnormal mitoses are more commonly seen in malignant cells.

mo-'dal-i-ty n. A cumbersome and imprecise word; in cancer treatment, used as therapeutic modality, meaning one of the several forms of treatment such as chemotherapy, surgical removal, or radiation treatment.

mu-'ta-tion n. 1. Alteration of a chromosome by physical or chemical process, which results in a continuously inherited change in the cells or organisms descended from that cell; example is mutation of a normal cell to a malignant cell. 2. Visible or identifiable change in the body, appearance, or function of a living organism, apparent from birth, resulting from alteration in the genetic material as in (1).

'ne-o-plasm n. (From Greek, "new growth.") (Adj., neoplastic.) A tumor; the words are essentially synonymous. As with tumor, may be either benign or malignant in its behavior.

on-'col-o-gist n. (Derived from oncology, the study of tumors.) A physician who specializes in the study and treatment of cancer; applied particularly to medical oncologists, who specialize primarily in chemotherapy of cancer. May also apply to other specialties, such as radiation oncologist, and surgical oncologist.

'pal-li-a-tion n. (Adj., palliative.) Relief of symptoms, such as pain or disability; the objective of cancer treatment when cure is not possible.

Pap smear n. (After the originator of the examination technique, Dr. George N. Papanicolaou [1883–1962], professor of pathology at Cornell University Medical College, New York.) A diagnostic technique by which body fluids or secretions may be spread on a glass slide, stained, and examined for the presence of malignant cells. First used to examine secretions from the uterine cervix; now used also to examine sputum, bronchial washings, pleural fluid, and others.

performance status n. Measure of activity of which a cancer patient is capable, noting in order: absence of symptoms; symptoms but ability to maintain full activity; ability to maintain limited activity; ability to care for self without assistance; proportion of the day spent in bed; need for continuous care; or finally moribund state. A good performance status tends to be associated with better response to treatment, especially to chemotherapy.

pe-'riph-er-y n. (Adj., peripheral.) In medicine, the outer portion of a limb, an organ, and so on, the area farthest from the center; in the lung, the area farthest out away from the hilum. In the periphery of the lung, the pulmonary arteries, veins, and bronchi have divided into their smallest branches.

'phe-no-type n. In cancer biology, the visible characteristics and behavior of a cell, or a cell line, by which its malignant or benign character may be established.

'pleu-ral spaces adj. and n. (Pronounced like plural). Two large spaces (right and left) within the chest cavity which contain the right and left lungs. Both spaces are lined with a fine smooth glistening membrane, the pleura.

'pleu-ri-sy n. Inflammation of the pleural surfaces, with resulting pain on moving or coughing, and accumulation of fluid in the pleural space; until thirty to forty years ago pleurisy usually was a sign of tuberculosis but this is relatively rare now. In this context, more likely to be used as malignant pleurisy, the involvement of pleural surfaces by tumor, again with pain, fluid accumulation, and increasing shortness of breath.

pneu-mo-'nec-tom-y n. (Initial letter "p" is silent.) Surgical removal of an entire lung, usually for cancer; may be left or right. Differentiated from *lobectomy*, removal of a lobe, an operation of lesser magnitude and hence preferable when it will adequately remove the disease.

'pol-yp n. (Adj., *polypoid*, in the form of a polyp.) A small tumorlike growth in the membrane lining the intestine, somewhat in the form of a puffball mushroom but usually with a longer stalk; ordinarily benign but with the potential of becoming malignant.

primary tumor adj. and n. Tumor that grows at the place where the first malignant change of a cell occurred, at the primary site; differentiated from the *metastases*, or secondary tumors, which appear as a result of spread away from the primary.

pro-phy-'lac-tic adj. (From Greek, "guarding against, beforehand.") When used in regard to treatment, denotes treatment aimed to prevent some adverse occurrence from happening; as, prophylactic radiation therapy to the brain in treatment of small-cell carcinoma of the lung, to prevent appearance of brain metastases.

pro-'spec-tive adj. (From Latin, "looking forward.") In medicine, a study or clinical trial which has been defined and planned before it is conducted, so that all subjects meet specified requirements; as opposed to retrospective, a study that evaluates treatment given in the past, which usually had not been in accordance with a plan.

'pro-to-col n. In this context, a formal, detailed plan for treatment of a given tumor type; often an experimental treatment, in which case the plan must have prior approval from the institutional review board, and the patient must give special and detailed permission for the treatment plan to be carried out.

'prox-i-mal adj. In anatomy, refers to the portion of a limb, an organ, etc., which is closest to the center (of the body); the opposite of *distal*.

'pul-mo-na-ry insufficiency n. (Pulmonary: pertaining to the lungs.) Inability of the lungs to adequately perform their function, respiratory gas exchange, by reason of disease or anatomic changes; therefore, a syndrome or clinical state of chronically feeling short of breath, "unable to get enough air," inability to perform any exertion.

ra-di-'og-raph-y n. (Adj., *radiographic*). The method or system of forming images of the body's interior from X-ray beams, for diagnostic purposes.

râles plural n. (Rhymes with shalls). Fine crackling sounds which may be heard in the lung during breathing, by means of a stethoscope; abnormal when present, in that they suggest fluid retention within the lung, "wet lung." When râles are absent, the breath sounds are said to be clear.

'ran-dom-ized adj. When applied to research studies, clinical trials of new drugs or treatment, specifies that the patients or the subjects were assigned to one or the other treatment in a truly random manner, so that bias or selection are eliminated from the study.

re-'gress-ion n. In this context, diminution in size or disappearance of a cancer; may result from chemotherapy or irradiation, as partial or as complete regression; or rarely, may occur without known cause, as spontaneous regression.

re-'sec-tion n. Applied principally to the gastrointestinal tract and the lungs, surgical removal of part or all of an organ; such as gastric resection, colon resection, pulmonary resection. When other organs are removed, the procedure is called excision.

'ret-i-noids plural n. (See also *carotenoids*.) A group of biochemical compounds, Vitamin A and its synthetic analogues; under investigation for possible cancer-preventive effects.

sar-'com-a n. A malignant tumor, differentiated from *carcinoma* by its origin not from epithelial or surface-lining cells, but from the cells of muscle, connective tissue, bone, and so on. Behavior of sarcomas differs from that of carcinomas in certain ways; but both fall under the loose meaning of the popular term *cancer*, a malignant tumor of any kind.

'seg-ment n. When applied to the lung, a subdivision of a lobe; a lobe has from two to five segments. An individual segment can be removed surgically (segmental resection); but in treatment of lung cancer, this is done only if the tumor is very small, located in the periphery of the lung, and there is need to preserve as much of the patient's lung tissue as possible.

se-'nes-cence n. The process of aging, growing old; applicable to cells and tissues as well as to individuals.

small-cell carcinoma n. (More properly, small-cell undifferentiated carcinoma). One of the histologic types of primary lung cancer; the fastest growing and the most malignant of all in its biologic behavior; heavily dependent on smoking history. This particular tumor type ordinarily cannot be treated effectively by surgical removal, because it is almost always widespread when first discovered. It responds, often dramatically, to treatment by radiotherapy and chemotherapy, but is seldom cured.

specimen n. In surgery, the organ or tissue removed by excision, or by biopsy; it must be forwarded to the pathologist for careful examination including microscopic sections, which are the basis for the pathologist's report. In lung cancer surgery, the specimen is the lobe or lung removed as treatment, together with its lymph nodes.

'squam-ous cells adj. and n. Thin flattened cells arranged in a layer covering certain body surfaces, particularly skin surface, mucous membranes lining the mouth, tongue, and so on. In the context of this volume, the cell of origin of squamous-cell carcinoma, one of the commonest types of primary lung cancer.

stage n. Applied to malignant tumors, a measure of how far the disease has progressed, therefore in general terms a determinant of prognosis after treatment. Staging rules vary with each type of malignancy. Without thorough knowledge of tumor types, biologic behavior, and results of therapy, any detailed outline of staging criteria is likely only to bewilder and mislead the reader.

'syn-drome n. (From Greek, "concurrence.") A complex or a set of symptoms that occur together, not constituting a specific disease but more loosely, a morbid state. In this volume, refers especially to the para-neoplastic syndromes which may occur as a secondary effect in a few cases of lung cancer. ("Para-neoplastic": designating the complex of symptoms other than those characteristically caused by tumor itself.)

'syn-ge-'ne-ic adj. (From Greek, "having closely related genes.") Animals belonging to a strain so highly inbred that their genetic compositions are for practical purposes the same. As a result individuals will accept tissue or organ grafts from each other without suppressive treatment. Not quite the same as *isogeneic*, individuals born with identical genetic composition, as human identical twins.

tho-'rac-ic adj. (Rhymes with name of the geological period, Jurassic). From Greek and Latin thorax, the chest. Pertaining to, or having to do with, the chest; in this volume usually appearing as thoracic surgery, surgery of the chest that is concerned primarily with the heart, lungs, esophagus, etc.

'trac-he-a n. The "windpipe," or single passageway through which air passes to and from both lungs during respiration; the trachea ends at its point of division, or bifurcation, into the two main bronchi.

'tra-che-'ost-omy n. (From Greek, the making of an orifice into the trachea.) An opening, or window, in the trachea in the lower neck anteriorly, allowing a silver or plastic tube to pass into the trachea and thus to serve as a new, shorter airway for breathing. Properly spelled with an "s," signifying a *stoma* or opening into the trachea; the older and less accurate spelling tracheotomy signifies only cutting into the trachea (Greek *tomos*, a cutting instrument). Tracheostomy is most often used today to allow assisted breathing by a mechanical ventilator, or to bypass obstruction of the airway.

'tum-or n. An independent "new growth," resulting from genetic change in a cell which removes biologic controls on its continued growth and multiplication. May be benign (slowly growing, non-invasive, non-spreading; hence unlikely to be fatal to the host), or malignant (more rapidly growing, invasive, able to spread; hence potentially fatal to the host). Malignant tumors are commonly known as cancers; the terms are essentially synonymous.

un-dif-fer-'en-ti-a-ted adj. (See also *anaplastic*.) Applied principally to malignant tumors; usually modifies the noun identifying a more specific cell type. Designates malignant tumors made up of, or containing, primitive unspecialized cells; often with much variation between cells; likely to be more malignant in its behavior than one made up of more mature, specialized, or differentiated cells.

'ver-te-brae plural n.; (singular, *vertebra*) The bones of the spinal column, somewhat in the shape of spools stacked upon each other; each bone has an arch-shaped structure posteriorly which covers and protects the spinal cord. Twelve vertebrae have attached ribs and are called the thoracic vertebrae.

'vol-vu-lus n. Applied principally to the intestinal tract; a twisting of a portion of the intestine with the result that it is not only obstructed, but its blood supply may be cut off; likely to be fatal unless promptly relieved by surgery.

Index

Page numbers in boldface refer to items in the Glossary; page numbers in italics refer to figures.

chromosome, **215**; genetic information in, 45
Churchill, Winston, 129
cigarette manufacturers: liability of, 134–138; yearly after-tax profits of, *138*
cigarettes: addiction to, 97, 98, 139–143; advertising for, 4, 155–158, 159–160; annual per capita consumption of, 156; chemical analysis of tobacco in, 21; "low-yield," 20–21, 140; package warnings for, 154; taxes on, 154–155; withdrawal reactions to, 140–141
cigarette smoke, second-hand, 19–20, 100
cigarette smoking: developing habit of, 1–8; at early age, 42–43; economic sanctuary for, 158–159; effects of quitting, 16–17; glamorous image of, 159–160; in larynx cancer, 93; link of to lung cancer, 4, 9–10, 15–19, 58–59; public weal and, 153–155; religious or ethical prohibition of, 21–22; treatment programs for dependence on, 141–143; in women, 12
Cipollone, Rose, 135–138
Cipollone v. *Liggett Group, Lorillard Inc. and Philip Morris Inc.*, 135–136
cis-diammine-dichloro-platinum, 84
cisplatin, 84, 88, 126
Clarke, Arthur C., 161, 183
cobalt mining, 22, 125
cocaine, 141
coin lesions, 63–64; prompt removal of, 115; X-ray of, 189–192
colorectal carcinoma, **215**; diet and, 26
Committee for Freedom of Choice in Cancer Therapy, Inc., 149
computerized tomographic (CT) scan, 34, **215**; of chest, 195–199; in diagnosis, 63
Constitution, U.S., 153
coping, 53–59
cosmos, as blind machine, 56
coughing, 28, 98–99; with blood-streaked sputum, 93–94; as early symptom, 48

cryoablation, 37
cryolysis, 73
curability factors, 113–121
cyclophosphamide (Cytoxan), 83, 88, 124, 126
cytological studies, 47; of sputum, 61–63
cytology, **215**

Daynard, Richard, 135
death, reality of, 56
Death in the West, 159
DeBakey, Dr. Michael, 10
Decadron pills, 94
defense mechanisms, 55–56
delta-9-tetra-hydro-cannabinol, 25
density, radiographic, 183
deoxyribonucleic acid (DNA) strands, 45
dependence, 141
detoxification treatment, 148
diagnosis, 60–66
diaphragm, **215**; functions of, 67–68
diet, lung cancer and, 26–27
dissemination, **215**
distal position, **215**
Doll, Dr. Richard, 15–16
Donne, John: on death, 28, 89; on effects of diagnosis, 60; on self-destructiveness, 9
doubling time, 169–177; formula for, 174; hypothesis of, 170–172; measurement and calculation in, 172–177
Douglas, Sen. Paul, 148
doxorubicin (Adriamycin), 84, 126
drugs, testing effectiveness of, 14–15
Durovic, Dr. Stevan, 148

economics, cigarette advertising and, 158–159
Edell, Marc Z., 137
Ehrlich, Dr. Paul, 83
emphysema, **215**
empyema, 75, **216**
endometrial cancer, 90
endometriosis, **216**
endotracheal tube, 69; respiration through, 70